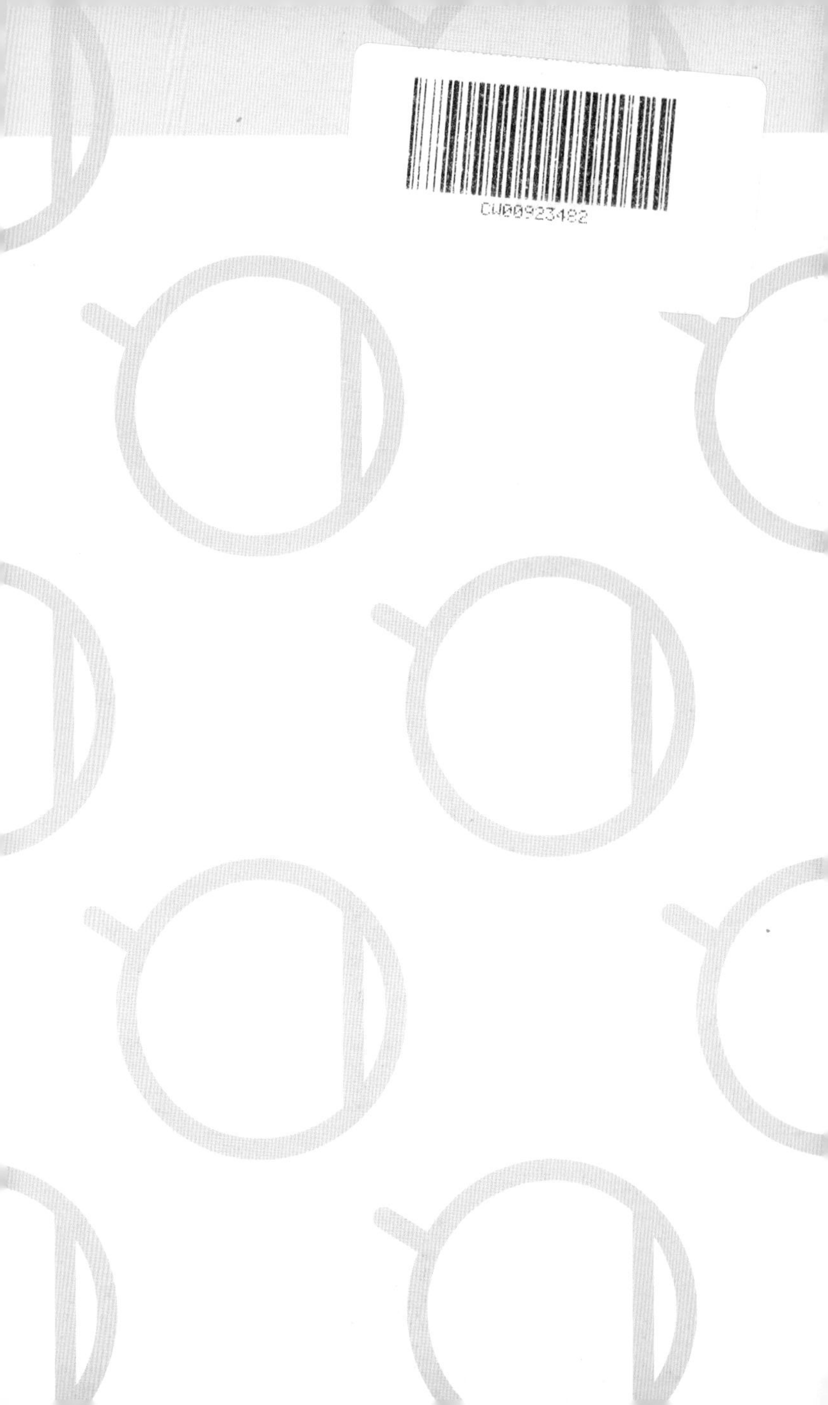
CW00923482

For Elsevier Butterworth-Heinemann:

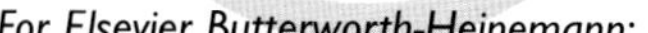

Publishing Director: Caroline Makepeace
Commissioning Editor: Robert Edwards
Development Editor: Kim Benson
Production Manager: Anne Dickie
Design Direction: George Ajayi

eye essentials

visual fields

Robert P Cubbidge PGCertHE, PhD, MCOptom
Lecturer, Optometry & Vision Sciences,
School of Life & Health Sciences, Aston University,
Birmingham, UK

SERIES EDITORS
Sandip Doshi PhD, MCOptom
Optometrist in private practice, Hove, East Sussex, UK
Examiner, College of Optometrists, London, UK
Formerly Clinical Editor, Optician Journal

William Harvey MCOptom
Visiting Clinician and Director of Visual Impairment Clinic,
City University, London, UK
Professional Programme Tutor for Boots Opticians Ltd
Clinical Editor, Optician Journal, Reed Business Information, Sutton, UK

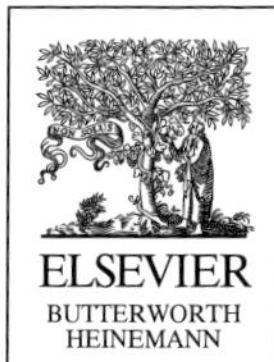

EDINBURGH LONDON NEW YORK OXFORD
PHILADELPHIA ST LOUIS SYDNEY TORONTO 2005

ELSEVIER
BUTTERWORTH
HEINEMANN

First published 2005

ISBN 0 7506 8851 3

British Library Cataloguing in Publication Data
A catalogue record for this book is available from the British Library.

Library of Congress Cataloging in Publication Data
A catalog record for this book is available from the Library of Congress.

Note
Knowledge and best practice in this field are constantly changing. As new research and experience broaden our knowledge, changes in practice, treatment and drug therapy may become necessary or appropriate. Readers are advised to check the most current information provided (i) on procedures featured or (ii) by the manufacturer of each product to be administered, to verify the recommended dose or formula, the method and duration of administration, and contraindications. It is the responsibility of the practitioner, relying on their own experience and knowledge of the patient, to make diagnoses, to determine dosages and the best treatment for each individual patient, and to take all appropriate safety precautions. To the fullest extent of the law, neither the publisher nor the editors assumes any liability for any injury and/or damage to persons or property arising from this publication.

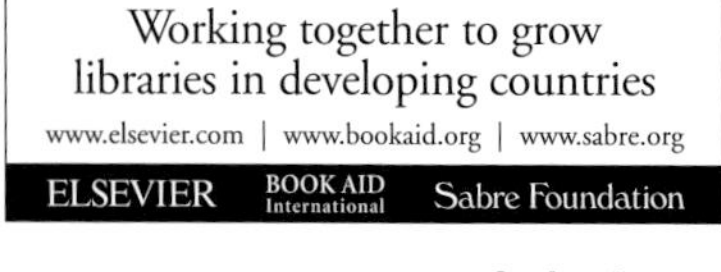

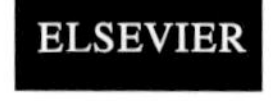

your source for books, journals and multimedia in the health sciences

www.elsevierhealth.com

The publisher's policy is to use **paper manufactured from sustainable forests**

Printed in China

Contents

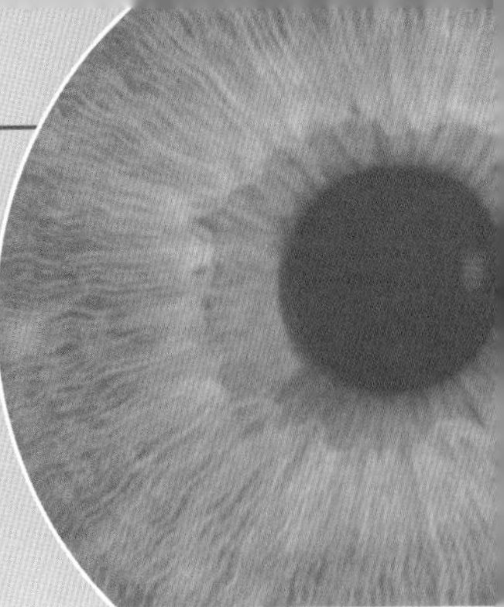

Foreword

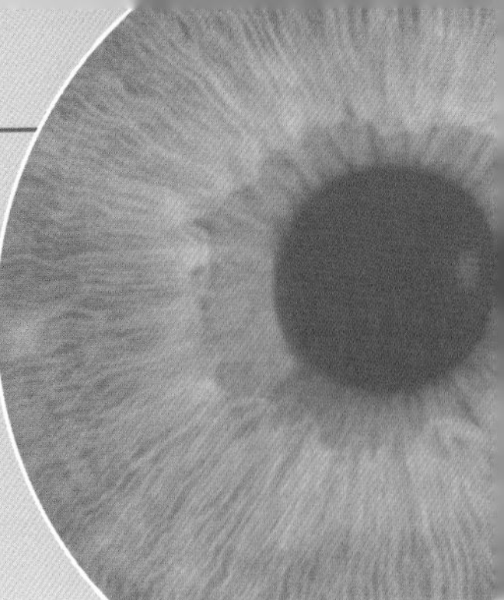

Eye Essentials is a series of books intended to cover the core skills required by the eye care practitioner in general and/or specialized practice. It consists of books covering a wide range of topics, ranging from: routine eye examination to assessment and management of low vision; assessment and investigative techniques to digital imaging; case reports and law to contact lenses.

Authors known for their interest and expertise in their particular subject have contributed books to this series. The reader will know many of them, as they have published widely within their respective fields. Each author has addressed key topics in their subject in a practical rather than theoretical approach, hence each book has a particular relevance to everyday practice.

Each book in the series follows a similar format and has been designed to enable the reader to ascertain information easily and quickly. Each chapter has been produced in a user-friendly format, thus providing the reader with a rapid-reference book that is easy to use in the consulting room or in the practitioner's free time.

Optometry and dispensing optics are continually developing professions, with the emphasis in each being redefined as we learn more from research and as technology stamps its mark. The *Eye Essentials* series is particularly relevant to the practitioner's requirements and as such will appeal to students, graduates sitting professional examinations and qualified practitioners alike. We hope you enjoy reading these books as much as we have enjoyed producing them.

Sandip Doshi
Bill Harvey

1
Introduction

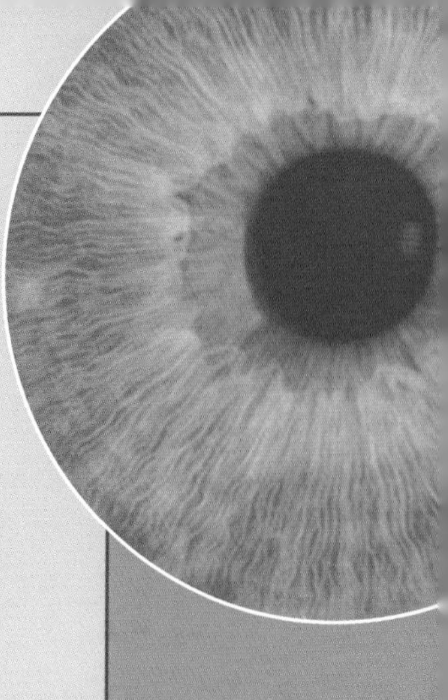

The clinical visual field is best defined as *all the space an eye can see at any given instant in time.* The monocular dimensions of the visual field in an average person extend to 60 degrees superiorly and 70 degrees inferiorly. Horizontally, the nasal visual field extends to 60 degrees and 100 degrees temporally. These dimensions are, of course, approximate and are limited by an individual's facial anatomy; primarily the frontal, maxillary, nasal and zygomatic bones. Eyelid position, hairstyle, the prominence of the eyebrows and the nose can also limit the visual field. Binocularly, the two monocular visual fields overlap, resulting in a stereoscopic zone which is approximately 120 degrees in the horizontal dimension. The extreme temporal periphery of the binocular field is seen monocularly. The retinal image of the visual field is upside down and back to front. Therefore, the projection of the visual field is such that the superior visual field corresponds to the inferior retina and vice-versa. Similarly, the temporal component of the visual field corresponds to the nasal retina and vice-versa.

Classically, the visual field has been likened to an island of vision surrounded by a sea of blindness. The hill of vision is a three-dimensional representation of retinal light sensitivity. Using this concept, it becomes easier to visualize changes in light sensitivity which occur in the different patterns of visual field loss (Figure 1.1). The sea represents those areas of the visual field where there is no light perception, for example, the visual field which is invisible due to the anatomical limits of the face. There is a gradual rise in altitude of the island, culminating at a peak at its center, which represents the increasing sensitivity to light from the retinal periphery to the fovea. Under photopic conditions, the shape of the hill of vision is closely correlated to the packing density of cones and receptive field size. The greatest packing density of cones occurs at the fovea, where cones average approximately 16,000 cones/deg^2 and decreases sharply towards the retinal periphery, where the density is approximately 300 cones/deg^2 at 32 degrees eccentricity. Similarly, receptive field size is much smaller in the central retina than in the periphery. Cone density does not decrease across the retina linearly, with the result that the sensitivity of gradient hill of vision is steeper

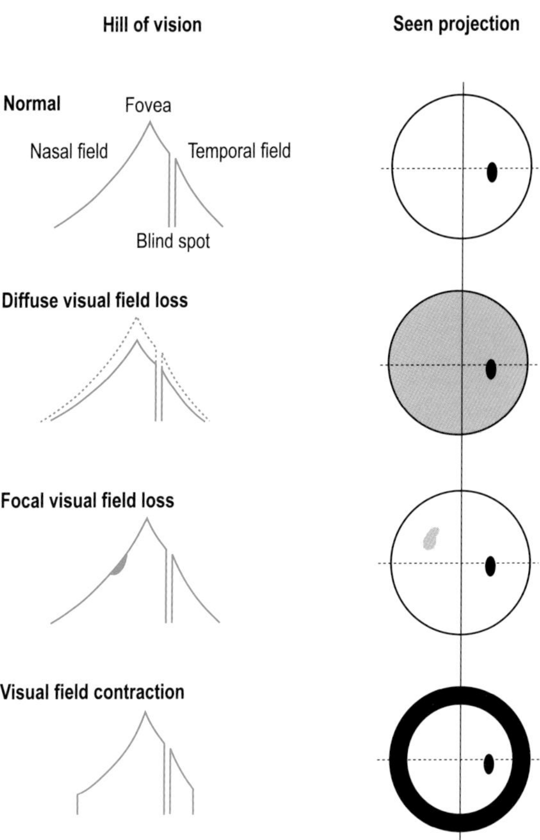

Figure 1.1 The hill of vision representation and the seen projection of the visual field (right eye)

nasally than temporally and steeper superiorly than inferiorly. With increasing age, the hill of vision reduces in height and its slopes become steeper. In part, this is due to the reduction in retinal luminance, induced by a reduction in the transmission of the ocular media and pupil size. The greatest contribution to the age-related reduction in the height of the hill of vision is thought to derive from the decline in photoreceptors, retinal neurones and pigment epithelial cells.

A visual field defect is defined as any departure from the normal topography of the hill of vision. Pre-retinal opacities, such as corneal lesion, age-related cataract and other media opacities scatter light and reduce light transmission through the eye, thereby reducing sensitivity to light evenly across the visual field. This causes a generalized reduction in the height of the hill of vision; a type of visual field loss called a depression or, more commonly, diffuse visual field loss (Figure 1.1). Diseases which damage the peripheral retina, such as retinitis pigmentosa, glaucoma and the toxic effects of some drugs, cause the circumference of the island of vision to reduce at sea level. Such a loss in the peripheral margins of the visual field is termed a contraction (Figure 1.1).

Non-uniform reduction in light sensitivity in the visual field is called focal loss (Figure 1.1). An area of reduced light sensitivity surrounded by an area of normal sensitivity, is called a relative scotoma. Where there is no light perception in an area surrounded by normal sensitivity, the scotoma is termed absolute. The physiological blind spot is an example of an absolute scotoma.

Useful Reading

Atchison, D.A. (1979). History of visual field measurement. *Aust. J. Optom.* **62**: 345–354.

Aulhorn, E. and Harms, H. (1972). Visual perimetry. Visual psychophysics: *Handbook of sensory physiology*. Eds: Jameson, D. and Hurvich, L.M. Springer-Verlag, Berlin, VII. pp. 102–145.

Curcio, C.A. and Sloan, K.R. (1992). Packing geometry of human cone photoreceptors: variation with eccentricity and evidence for local anisotropy. *Vis. Neurosci.* **9**: 169–180.

Gao, H. and Hollyfield, J.G. (1992). Aging of the human retina. *Invest. Ophthalmol. Vis. Sci.* **33**: 1–17.

Heijl, A., Lindgren, G. and Olsson, J. (1987). Normal variability of static perimetric threshold values across the central visual field. *Arch. Ophthalmol.* **105**: 1544–1549.

2 Classification and localization of visual field defects

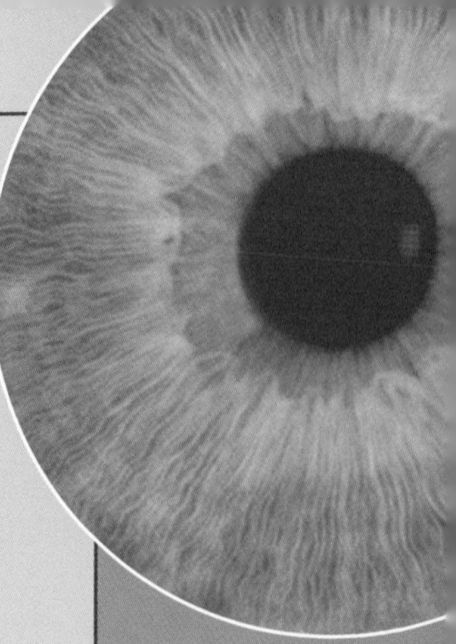

The blind spot is approximately 7.5 degrees high and 5.5 degrees wide and represents the temporal visual field projection of the optic nerve, found approximately 1.5 degrees below and 15 degrees horizontally from fixation. When interpreting visual field defects knowledge of the arrangement of nerve fibers in visual pathway is essential.

Depending on the site of damage in the visual pathway, characteristic visual field defects are produced (Figure 2.1).

Retina

Anatomically, the visual pathway begins at the photoreceptors which lie in the outer retina. Here, photons of light are absorbed by the photopigments, which are sensitive to specific regions of the visible electromagnetic spectrum. Light energy is converted into electrical signals, which are conveyed along the visual pathway. Should photoreceptors lose sensitivity, a scotoma would form in the visual field. As the density profile of photoreceptors varies from the center to peripheral retina, scotomas would be expected to be larger in the periphery of the visual field than in the center. Damage to the photoreceptors and choroid can occur in a variety of ways; laser photocoagulation scars, chorioretinal inflammations and degenerations, drug induced toxicities affecting photoreceptor physiology, and vascular damage occurring within the inner retina. The resulting scotomas usually occur monocularly and would not respect the horizontal and vertical midlines of the visual field. Scotomas which form within a radius 30 degrees from the fovea are termed paracentral scotomas.

The inner retina consists of the retinal nerve fiber layer, which follows a characteristic pattern as it passes towards the optic nerve (Figure 2.2). The inferior and superior nerve fibers do not cross the horizontal midline of the retina, thereby forming a line of demarcation passing though the fovea, called the horizontal raphé. Nerve fibers in the macular area, which travel to the optic nerve, form the papillomacular bundle. Those inferior and superior temporal fibers which do not form the papillomacular bundle arch around it as they travel to the optic nerve. Inferior

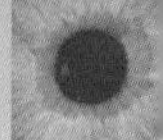

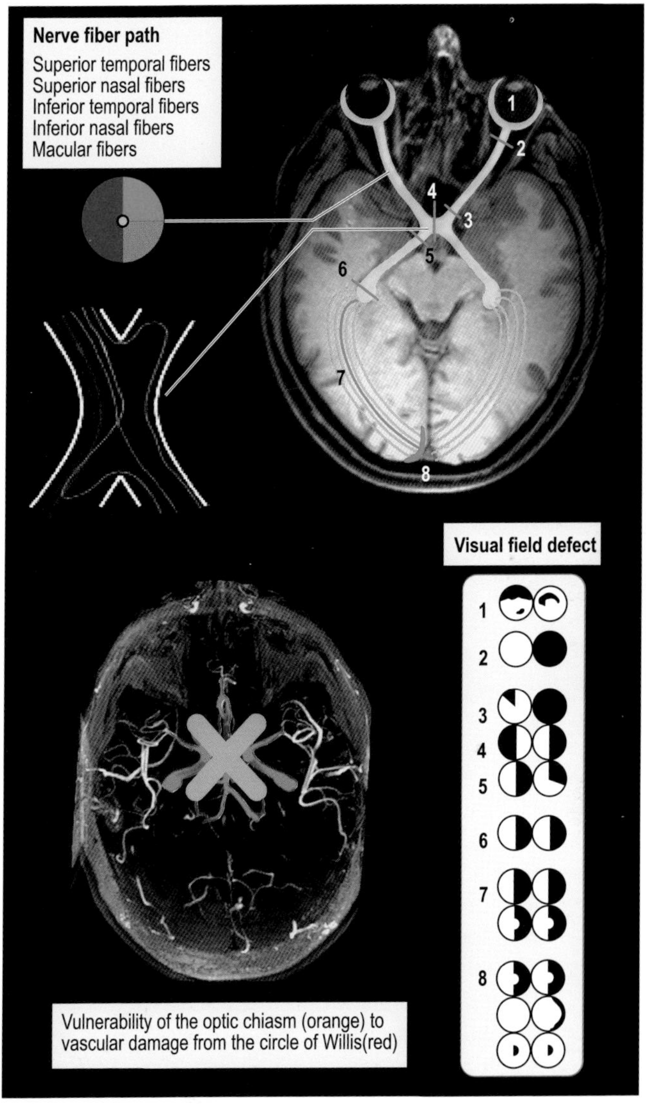

Figure 2.1 The visual pathway and its associated visual field

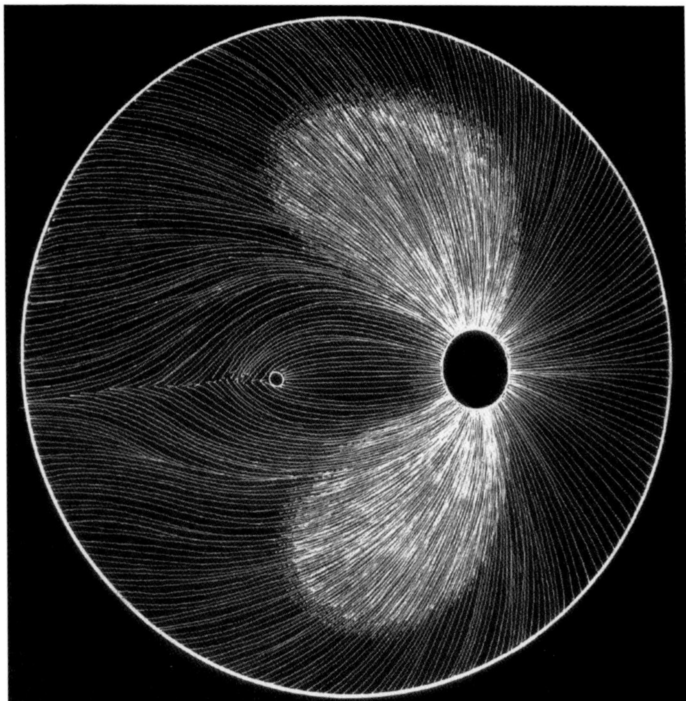

Figure 2.2 Distribution of retinal nerve fibers. Reproduced from Litwak, *Glaucoma handbook* (2000, Butterworth-Heinemann) with permission

and superior nasal fibers follow a more direct course to the optic nerve as they are not hindered by the papillomacular bundle. The nerve fibers from the nasal retina do not cross those of the temporal retina and thereby form a theoretical vertical line of demarcation, which passes through the center of the fovea. Damage to the retinal nerve fibers gives rise to characteristic arcuate scotomas. Damage to the vascular supply of the inner retina, resulting from branch retinal artery and vein occlusion, will typically give rise to large scotomas which are altitudinal in shape (loss in the upper or lower half of the visual field with a sharply defined horizontal border). If a scotoma forms within the papillomacular nerve fiber bundle and is continuous with the

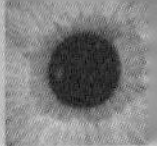

physiological blind spot, the visual field defect is described as a centrocaecal scotoma. Scotomas of the papillomacular nerve fiber bundle which are not continuous with the blind spot are described as central scotomas.

Optic nerve

The retinal nerve fibers exit the retina via the optic nerve head. Diseases which affect the optic nerve head give rise to visual field defects, which are determined by the path of the retinal nerve fiber layer. A number of conditions affect the optic nerve, including glaucoma, anterior ischaemic optic neuropathy, papilloedema and thyroid optic neuropathy. The formation of a large arcuate scotoma, which extends to the horizontal raphé, will lead to an area in the nasal visual field which has reduced light sensitivity on one side of the horizontal raphé and normal sensitivity on the other. This type of defect is called a nasal step and is one of the characteristic features of visual field loss in glaucoma. Congenital abnormalities of the optic nerve head, such as optic pits, tilted discs and optic nerve head drusen may yield arcuate scotomas and nasal steps.

Once the nerve fibers leave the eye and pass into the optic nerve, damage to the visual pathway is not visible with an ophthalmoscope and, in an optometric practice, is only detectable by visual field examination. Reorganization of the nerve fibers takes place along the entire length of the visual pathway and, consequently, the shape of the resulting visual field defect can be used to identify the location of damage in the visual pathway, which is often a result of mechanical compression of the nerve fibers or vascular damage. At the level of the lamina cribrosa, the nerve fibers have the same orientation as the optic nerve head. A short distance after leaving the optic nerve head, the fibers reorganize and the macular fibers pass towards the center of the optic nerve. Inferior and superior temporal fibers locate to the inferior and superior temporal aspect of the nerve respectively and, similarly, inferior and superior nasal fibers locate towards the inferior and superior nasal aspect.

Optic chiasm

At the optic chiasm, approximately 50% of the nasal nerve fibers, including the nasal macular fibers, cross into the contralateral optic tract. Many of the inferior nasal fibers pass backwards into the optic nerve before looping back and crossing the chiasm, passing into the contralateral optic tract. These looping fibers form the anterior knees of Wilbrand. The posterior knees of Wilbrand are formed by the superior nasal fibers (including the temporal macular fibers) passing into the ipsilateral optic tract, before looping back and crossing the chiasm, passing into the contralateral optic tract. Temporal nerve fibers do not cross at the optic chiasm and pass through the temporal aspect of the chiasm into the ipsilateral optic tracts (Figure 2.3). The optic chiasm is particularly vulnerable to compressive and vascular damage, as it lies above the pituitary gland and is also encased by the circle of Willis, a vascular structure in the base of the cranial cavity.

The circle of Willis represents the entry point into the cranial cavity of the major blood supply to the cerebrum. The carotid

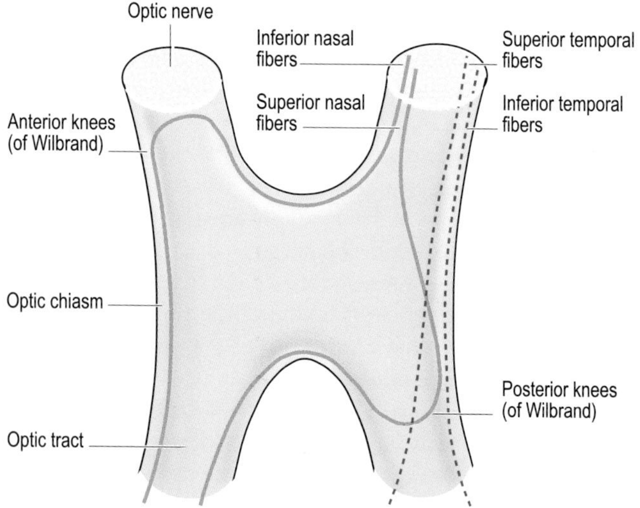

Figure 2.3 Optic chiasm

artery presents a direct pathway into the brain from embolisms originating in the neck and is consequently a common site of stroke. Hemorrhages or aneurysms of the carotid artery in the circle of Willis cause compression of the lateral aspect of the optic chiasm, resulting in damage to the superior and inferior temporal fibers (see Figure 2.1). The corresponding visual field defect would be a unilateral nasal hemianopia (loss of one half of the visual field, respecting the vertical midline), the eye indicating the same side of the optic chiasm affected. Occasionally, an aneurysm may cause so much compression that it displaces the optic chiasm against the corresponding carotid artery on the opposite side of the chiasm. This would result in a bilateral nasal hemianopia. When hemianopias and quadrantanopias (visual field loss in a quadrant, respecting the horizontal and vertical midlines) form bilaterally, they are further classified either homonymous or heteronymous. In homonymous visual field defects, the hemianopia affects the same side of the visual field in both eyes, i.e. either both nasal visual fields, or both temporal visual fields. In heteronymous visual field defects, opposite sides of the visual field are affected, i.e. the temporal visual field of one eye and the nasal field of the other eye. Heteronymous visual field defects indicate that the site of damage has occurred at the optic chiasm. Homonymous visual field defects indicate that the site of damage to the visual pathway is either at the chiasm or posterior to it.

Inferior to the optic chiasm is the pituitary gland, located in the Sella Turcica, a bony cavity of the sphenoid bone. Tumors of the pituitary gland may expand upwards, leading to compression of the inferior aspect of the optic chiasm. In approximately 80% of the normal population, the optic chiasm lies directly above the Sella Turcica. In cases of pituitary tumor extending upwards through the Sella Turcica in this population, compression of the crossing inferior nasal fibers occurs, leading initially to a quadrantanopia in the upper temporal visual fields of both eyes, which gradually extends to form a hemianopia in the temporal visual fields of both eyes. Bitemporal quadrantanopias or hemianopias are indicative of visual field loss occurring at the optic chiasm, before the decussation of the nasal fibers has occurred. In 10% of normal individuals, the optic chiasm is located more anteriorly over the sella turcica (pre-fixed). In these cases, a pituitary tumor would compress the optic tracts first. In the remaining 10% of the normal population, the optic chiasm is located more posteriorly over the sella turcica (post-fixed), causing a pituitary tumor to compress the optic nerve. When a pituitary tumor enlarges upwards in pre- and post-fixed optic chiasms, a junctional scotoma would be expected to form.

Craniopharyngiomas are tumors which encroach on the optic chiasm superiorly and posteriorly, so that the superior nasal fibers are compressed. Typically, an inferior bitemporal quadrantanopia would result and, as the tumor progresses, would extend into the superior visual field, also resulting in a bitemporal hemianopia. Meningiomas are tumors which compress either the optic nerve or the optic chiasm. When compression occurs at the junction of the optic nerve and optic chiasm, the anterior knee of Wilbrand may become affected. The resulting visual defect is typically a central scotoma in one eye, resulting from compression of the macular fibers, accompanied by a peripheral, junctional scotoma in the contralateral eye.

Optic tract

Within the optic tracts further reorganization of the nerve fibers occurs. The distinction between nasal and temporal fibers is lost as they amalgamate together. The superior nerve fibers move towards the medial aspect of the optic tract and inferior fibers move towards the lateral aspect. The nerve fibers associated with the macular reorganize between the superior and inferior fibers. Lesions of the optic tracts are rare, but would be expected to produce a homonymous hemianopia or quadrantanopia, although junctional scotomas are possible if the site of the lesion is close to optic chiasm and interrupts the posterior knee of Wilbrand. When a homonymous defect affects the nasal visual field of the right eye and the temporal visual field of the left eye, the site of damage to the visual pathway will be beyond the chiasm on the right side. The opposite is true of lesions occurring beyond the optic chiasm on the left side.

LGN

The nerve fibers originating from the retina finally synapse with neurones projecting to the visual cortex at the lateral geniculate nucleus (LGN), a knee-shaped structure located in the dorsal lateral aspect of the thalamus. In cross section, the LGN consists of six layers, each receiving inputs from the various portions of the visual field (Figure 2.4). Nerve fibers originating from the inferior retinal quadrants synapse in the lateral aspect of the LGN, whilst those originating from the superior retinal quadrants synapse in the medial aspect. Macular fibers synapse in the triangular shaped wedge created between the superior and inferior fibers. Each of the layers within the LGN receives inputs from only one eye. Crossed nasal fibers synapse in layers 1, 4 and 6, whilst uncrossed temporal fibers terminate in the remaining layers (Figure 2.4).

Furthermore, fibers which carry signals that correspond to the same point in the visual field of both eyes are in alignment within each layer of the LGN, thus forming a retinotopic map which is a point-for-point localization of the retinal topography and, therefore, the visual field.

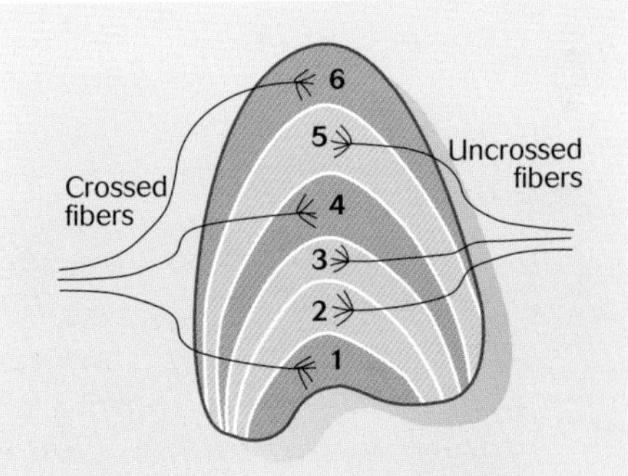

Figure 2.4 Six-layered structure of lateral geniculate nucleus showing the destination of crossed and uncrossed fibers. Reproduced from Doshi and Harvey, *Investigative Techniques and Ocular Examination* (2003, Butterworth-Heinemann) with permission

Congruence describes the degree of symmetry between two hemianopias or quadrantanopias. If the two hemianopias or quadrantanopias are superimposed on each other and the extent and shape of visual field defect matches exactly, the visual field defect is said to be congruent. When there is not a complete overlap, the defect is termed incongruent. The degree of congruence assists in the localization of the visual field defect in the visual pathway. Hemianopias and quadrantanopias which are incongruent occur before the LGN and the degree of congruence increases towards the striate cortex due to the formation of the retinotopic map.

Optic radiations

The nerve fibers leaving the LGN form the optic radiations in their route towards the striate cortex. Inferior nerve fibers representing the inferior retina leave the LGN and loop around the lateral ventricle passing towards the striate cortex, forming Meyer's loop (Figure 2.5).

Nerve fibers representing the superior retina form the superior radiations and follow a more direct path towards the striate cortex. Macular fibers pass to the striate cortex in a path

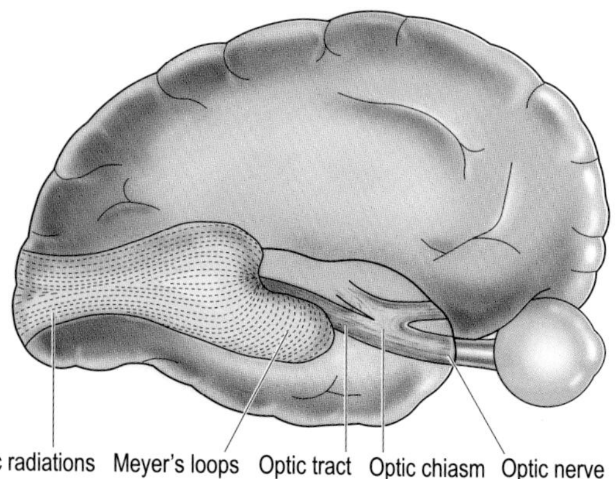

Figure 2.5 Meyer's Loop

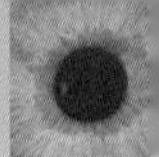

between the inferior and superior fibers. Lesions resulting in damage to the optic radiations are extremely rare and are most likely to occur as a result of damage to the vasculature in that area. Lesions resulting in damage to the superior optic radiations result in a homonymous defect which is inferior, quadrantic and wedge shaped, often termed "pie-on-the-floor". Conversely, damage to Meyer's loop leads to a homonymous, wedge shaped defect in the superior quadrants, often termed "pie in the sky".

Striate cortex

The inferior nerve fibers synapse in the lingual gyrus, which is an area of the striate cortex located just inferior to the calcarine fissure. Superior nerve fibers synapse in the cuneus gyrus, which is just superior to the calcarine fissure. Macular fibers synapse in the posterior-most region of the striate cortex. Macular fibers representing the inferior retina synapse in the lingual gyrus and superior macular fibers synapse in the cuneus gyrus. Retinotopic representation of the visual field is also present in the striate cortex, with the macular representation occupying a proportionately larger area than it does in the retina, as it is functionally more important to vision. Due to the high specialization of nerve fibers in the striate cortex, visual defects occurring at this site will exhibit a high degree of congruence. Vascular disease, strokes and mechanical trauma to the occipital region of the skull are the most common causes of visual field defects in the striate cortex. A number of unique hemianopias occur at the striate cortex, which include homonymous hemianopia, where the macular visual field is unaffected (macular sparing), or homonymous hemianopia affecting only the macular visual field (macular splitting).

Further Reading

Remington, L.A. and McGill, E.C. (1998). Clinical anatomy of the visual system. Boston, Oxford, Butterworth-Heinemann.

Kanski, J.J. (2003). Clinical ophthalmology, 5th Edition. Oxford, Butterworth-Heinemann.

3
Kinetic versus static perimetry

From Chapter 2 it can be seen that visual field defects manifest in a variety of retinal and neurological diseases. It is often recommended that visual field examination be carried out on any individual over the age of approximately 35. The basis of this recommendation is the increased incidence of glaucoma in patients over this age. Nevertheless, visual field defects commonly manifest in numerous other disease states, particularly those of neurological origin affecting the visual pathway. Such patients may present with symptoms such as headache or disturbed vision, but many of these conditions may be asymptomatic. Visual field examination is a straightforward and rapid procedure to carry out on the majority of patients and it should, therefore, be recommended that, in optometric practice, visual field examination be carried out on any patient who is capable of undergoing examination. The exact nature of the type of visual field examination to be carried out is dependent on the index of suspicion of finding a defect for a given patient. The index of suspicion is derived by the optometrist from the patient's history and from the clinical information obtained during an eye examination. In patients with a low index of suspicion, a fast screening procedure should be sufficient, whereas, in patients where there is an increased likelihood of eye or neurological disease, more sophisticated threshold visual field examinations should be considered.

Stimulus and background conditions for visual field examination

Perimetry is the measurement of the hill of vision in terms of establishing the patient's differential light sensitivity across the visual field. The normal shape of the hill of vision is dependent upon the state of retinal adaptation. Thus, in order to maintain consistent and reproducible results, the background illumination of any visual field examination must be carefully controlled. The majority of perimeters utilize a background luminance in the mesopic range, i.e. between 1 and 100 asb (the apostilb is the metric unit of light measurement employed in perimetry (1 asb = $1/\pi$ candelas m^{-2})). Additionally, the stimulus conditions must also be controlled for reproducible perimetry. During the 1930's, a Swiss ophthalmologist, Hans Goldmann, devised a series of circular light stimuli, which have been adopted as the standard for visual field examination. The smallest stimulus, Goldmann Size 0, has a diameter of 0.05° and area of 1/16 mm^2. Each successive stimulus size is twice the diameter (4 times the area) of the preceding stimulus, up to Goldmann Size V which has a diameter of 1.7° and an area of 64 mm^2. The standard stimulus size used in the majority of visual field examinations is a Goldmann Size III (0.43° diameter and area 4 mm^2).

Kinetic and static perimetry

Visual field examination can be accomplished by two methods; kinetic and static perimetry (Figure 3.1).

In kinetic perimetry, the patient fixates centrally and a stimulus, usually consisting of a circular self-luminous target or a patch of light, is slowly moved across the visual field from a non-seeing area until it is detected. It's location in the visual field is recorded by the examiner, who then presents the same stimulus at other positions in the visual field. Repeated measurements across the visual field enable the examiner to join the points of equal light sensitivity together, forming an isopter. In the normal eye, any point within an isopter is supraliminal, i.e. above threshold consciously perceived, unless the isopter encloses the

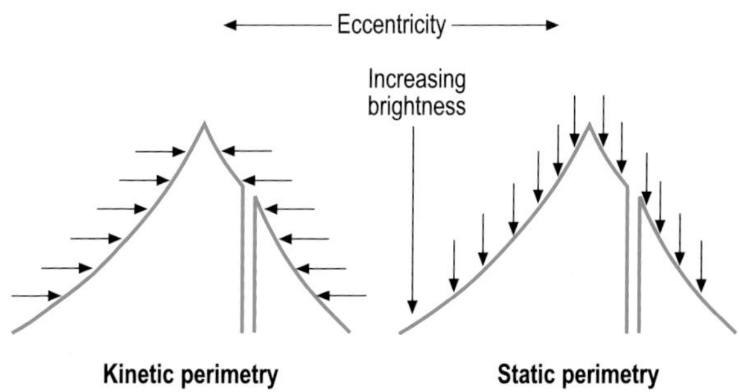

Figure 3.1 Kinetic and static perimetry

physiological blind spot. By using targets of different size and light intensity the examiner can construct a map of the visual field, which is analogous to looking at the height contours on a map. The optimal speed of movement of a kinetic stimulus is 4° per second. In its simplest form, kinetic perimetry can be accomplished using the confrontation test or gross perimetry (see Chapter 8).

Even when it is carried out under standardized stimulus and background conditions, the kinetic technique has been shown to suffer from a number of limitations. A moving stimulus will be detected more readily in the periphery than a static stimulus because of successive lateral spatial summation. As the stimulus moves across the visual field, spatial summation of receptive fields adjacent to the receptive field over which the stimulus is placed occurs. Thus, the detection of the stimulus will be influenced by normal areas of the visual field, in addition to any damaged areas, which could lead to shallow focal loss in the visual field being missed. More importantly, the position of the isopter is dependent upon the patient's reaction time to the detection of the stimulus and, additionally, the reaction time of the examiner in responding to the patient's response. The recent introduction of automated kinetic perimetry has standardized the stimulus velocity and eliminated the reaction time error of the examiner, but the visual field outcome is still influenced by the patient's reaction time and successive lateral summation. Despite these disadvantages, kinetic perimetry still has a place for the investigation of patients with profound visual field loss, as it can rapidly define areas of residual function and areas in the visual field with deep focal loss. It also remains the fastest method for delineating the limits of the visual field.

In static perimetry, light stimuli are presented in a fixed position in the visual field. In order to assess light sensitivity across the visual field, it is necessary to vary the intensity of the stimulus so that the threshold of light detection can be established. The size of the stimulus is constant and varied in intensity until the patient is just able to detect it. This point is called the threshold and represents the minimum light energy necessary to evoke a visual response with a probability of 0.5, i.e. the observer can detect the stimulus 50% of the time it is presented. A light stimulus presented below the threshold will not be detected by the observer, whereas a stimulus presented above the threshold will be detected by the observer. The threshold is expressed in terms of sensitivity, which is the reciprocal of the threshold. Sensitivity is presented in decibels (dB), which illustrates the logarithmic nature of light intensity on a linear scale. Decibels are calculated according to the following equation:

$$\text{Sensitivity (dB)} = \text{k} + \log\left(\frac{L}{\Delta L}\right)$$

Where k is a constant, L is the background luminance and ΔL is the stimulus luminance. 0 dB represents the brightest stimulus luminance of the perimeter. 1 dB is a 0.1 log unit reduction in intensity from the maximum stimulus luminance. 10 dB is equal to a 1 log unit reduction in intensity, 20 dB is equal to a 2 log unit reduction in intensity and 30 dB is equal to a 3 log unit reduction in intensity, representing 10, 100 and 1000 times attenuation in light intensity from the maximum stimulus luminance respectively. Because the decibel scale is dependent on the background luminance and the maximum stimulus is referenced to 0 dB, decibel scales are relative and will vary across perimeters, i.e. 30 dB on one perimeter is not the same as 30 dB on a different type of perimeter because the maximum stimulus luminance will be different across perimeter types.

The mode of stimulus presentation employed in static perimetry is governed by the purpose of the examination. Depending on whether the examination requires screening or accurate measurement, suprathreshold or full threshold examination may be undertaken (see next chapter).

Further Reading

Choplin, N.T., Sherwood, M.B. and Spaeth, G.L. (1990). The effect of stimulus size on the measured threshold values in automated perimetry. *Ophthalmology*. **97**, 371–374.

Fankhauser, F. (1986). Background illumination and automated perimetry. *Arch. Ophthalmol.* **104**, 1126.

Flanagan, J.G., Wild, J.M. and Hovis, J.K. (1991). The differential light threshold as a function of retinal adaptation- the Weber-Fechner / Rose-de-Vries controversy revisited. *Perimetry Update 1990/91*. RP Mills and A Heijl. Amsterdam/New York. Kugler Publications. 551–554.

Gilpin, L.B., Stewart, W.C., Hunt, H.H. and Broom, C.D. (1990). Threshold variability using different Goldmann stimulus sizes. *Acta Ophthalmol.* **68**: 674–676.

Sloan, L.L. (1961). Area and luminance of test object as variables in examination of the visual field by projection perimetry. *Vision Res.* **1**: 121–138.

4 Threshold strategies

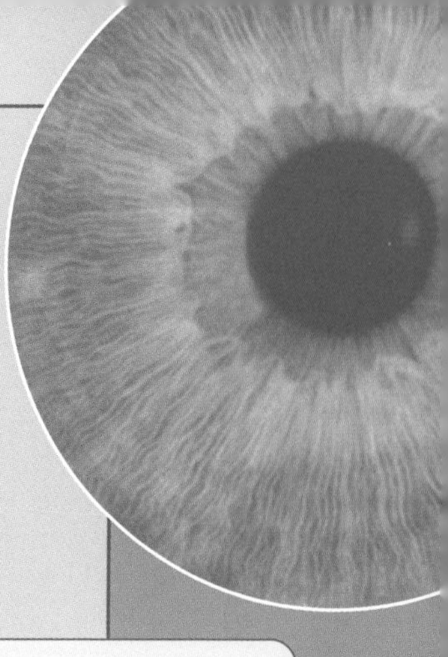

Suprathreshold strategy

In suprathreshold testing, the hill of vision is mapped at a stimulus level which is in the seeing region of the hill of vision, usually between 4 and 6 dB above the threshold (Figure 4.1). Suprathreshold examination offers a rapid examination of a large number of locations in the visual field. The ability of this technique to detect glaucoma is in the order of 90% or better. In its simplest form, a one level strategy, stimuli of constant luminance are presented at selected locations across the visual field (Figure 4.1). However, it is known that the hill of vision declines in sensitivity with increasing eccentricity from the fovea. It is, therefore, possible that a stimulus which is just suprathreshold in the periphery of the visual field may result in small relative defects being missed at the fovea or vice-versa (Figure 4.1). If the stimulus luminance is automatically modified to be brighter at more peripheral locations and dimmer centrally, the suprathreshold level will take into account the normal shape of the hill of vision and the technique will be yield equal sensitivity for scotoma detection across the visual field. In

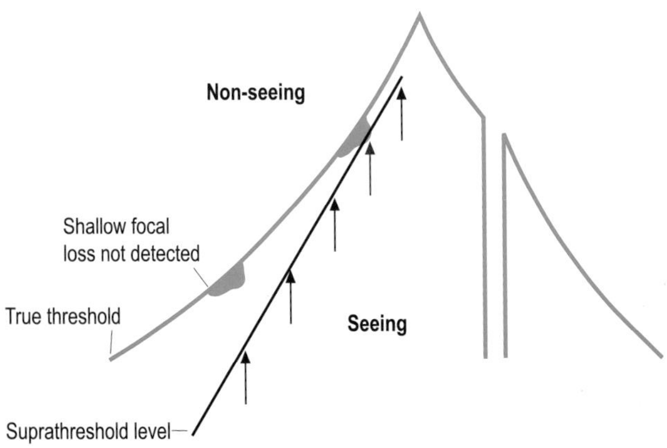

Figure 4.1 One-level suprathreshold strategy

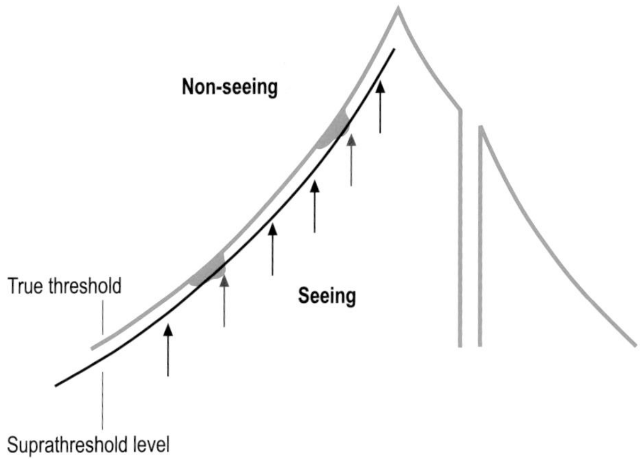

Figure 4.2 Gradient-adapted threshold strategy

consequence, adapting stimulus luminance across the hill of vision is more sensitive at defect detection than the one-level strategy. This approach is called a gradient-adapted suprathreshold strategy and is dependent upon knowledge of the hill of vision in a standard normal observer (Figure 4.2).

The disadvantage of employing a gradient-adapted approach is that the hill of vision exhibits considerable intra-individual variation in the normal observer, which can be as large as 10 dB, depending upon patient reliability and physiological factors. To account for this variation between normal individuals, a threshold-related gradient-adapted strategy, whereby the true threshold of the hill of vision is primarily obtained at a small number of central locations, is used in most modern perimeters, such as the Henson, Dicon and Humphrey series. The subsequent suprathreshold level of testing is selected on the basis of these initial thresholds. A further refinement to the threshold-related gradient-adapted suprathreshold method is to obtain the true threshold at all stimulus locations in the visual field where suprathreshold stimuli are not detected. Thus, where focal loss is detected with suprathreshold testing, the depth of visual field loss may also be quantified.

Full threshold strategy

The major disadvantage of suprathreshold visual field examination arises because it is testing at a stimulus level which is slightly above the threshold of light detection. Early and shallow focal loss which is of a depth between the estimated position of the hill of vision and the suprathreshold testing level will not be detected. Measuring the threshold at each stimulus location, instead of examining at suprathreshold level, will therefore be a more accurate measurement of the hill of vision. This technique is called full threshold static perimetry. It cannot be performed easily manually, and, therefore, is a feature of automated static perimetry. Until recently, it was extremely time consuming. Whereas a typical suprathreshold examination could take approximately 5 to 10 minutes to complete both eyes, a single full threshold examination of both eyes could take up to an hour. Historically, because of time pressures, optometrists in private practice in the UK predominantly employ the suprathreshold method for visual field examination and full threshold examination has largely been confined to hospital practice.

In a full threshold visual field examination, light sensitivity is determined at all stimulus locations in the visual field. The method of stimulus presentation in full threshold perimetry is called a staircase procedure. At a given location in the visual field, a stimulus of a particular brightness is presented to the observer. If the observer sees the stimulus they respond by pressing a button. The perimeter then reduces the light intensity of the stimulus by a predetermined step, e.g. 4 dB. Stimuli are presented in this manner until the observer does not detect the stimulus. At this point, the staircase has crossed the observer's threshold. Stimuli are then increased in smaller steps of brightness, e.g. 2 dB, until the patient detects the stimulus. In this case, the staircase has crossed the threshold twice and is recorded as the last seen stimulus. If the observer had not detected the first stimulus presented, the initial step size of the staircase would have traveled in the opposite direction, i.e. increased in 4 dB steps until detected and then reduced in 2 dB steps until not detected (Figure 4.3).

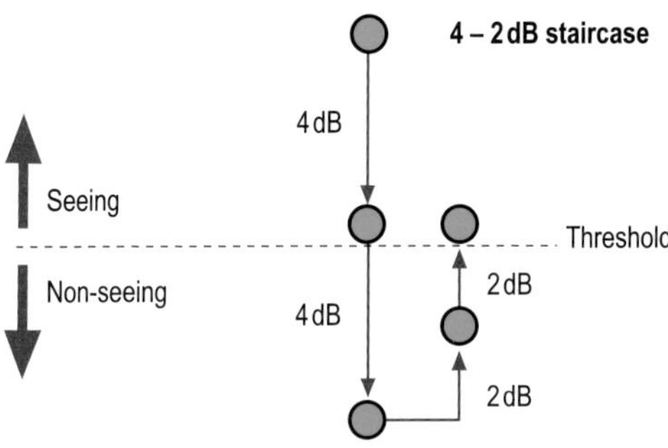

Figure 4.3 Full threshold staircase strategy

The physiological nature of the threshold is such that it varies from moment to moment and to a lesser degree from day to day. In perimetry, these variations in threshold are termed short- and long-term fluctuations. To measure the threshold with accuracy accounting for the short-term fluctuation, necessitates crossing the threshold many times. In psychophysics, staircases are designed so that the threshold is crossed many times, so that the threshold can be derived with great precision. In full threshold perimetry, because the threshold has to be determined at a large number of locations in the visual field, crossing the threshold many times is too time consuming. Thus, abbreviated staircases are employed where the threshold is crossed a maximum of two times at each location. This leads to a degree of imprecision in threshold determination such that the staircase procedure estimates the threshold rather than exactly finding its position. The threshold estimate is also, therefore, influenced by the short-term fluctuation. In full threshold perimetry, staircase procedures are employed using a pre-determined set of rules. This mode of threshold estimation is called an algorithm.

4-2 dB

Until recently, the most common threshold algorithm employed was the Full Threshold Algorithm, herewith termed the 4-2 dB algorithm. In the 4-2 dB algorithm, thresholds are estimated initially at four locations in the visual field, one in each quadrant at approximately nine degrees eccentricity from the fovea. The initial stimulus presentation of the staircase is determined from the observer's age. The initial step size used to vary stimulus brightness is 4 dB and, once the threshold is crossed, the step size is reduced to 2 dB steps. Stimulus presentation at the seed points occurs randomly, so that the position on the staircase is different for each location and the observer is not pre-conditioned to location of the next stimulus presentation. For the majority of perimeters the threshold is estimated as the last seen stimulus. Once the threshold has been estimated at a seed point, stimulus locations adjacent to the seed point are opened for threshold determination. At these locations, the initial stimulus presentation is at a brightness determined from the threshold previously obtained at the seed point.

Each subsequent threshold estimated opens up adjacent stimulus locations such that the order of stimulus presentation spirals out towards the visual field periphery. Because the smallest step size in the staircase is 2 dB, there will be a maximum error in threshold estimation of 2 dB. In the Octopus series of perimeters, a mathematical correction of 1 dB occurs between the last stimulus seen and not seen (a 4-2-1 dB staircase) in order to increase the precision of the estimate. Until recently, the 4-2 dB algorithm was recognized as the clinical "gold standard" for full threshold perimetry, since the short-term fluctuation is small and the results are highly reproducible. However, the large number of stimulus presentations required to estimate the thresholds across the visual field necessitated a long examination time (typically 12 minutes), requiring the observer to take regular breaks during the examination, which can lead to the results being influenced by observer concentration and fatigue.

FASTPAC

In an effort to reduce examination time, thereby minimizing fatigue and increasing observer vigilance, other staircase designs have been used for full threshold perimetry. The FASTPAC algorithm of the Humphrey series of perimeters utilizes a 3 dB step size and the staircase terminates when it has crossed the threshold once. Stimuli are initially presented in the predicted seeing region of the visual field at 50% of the locations tested and, for the remainder, the initial stimulus presentation is in the non-seeing region of the visual field. The threshold is recorded as the last seen stimulus, leading to an increase in the maximum error of threshold estimation to 3 dB over the 4-2 dB algorithm. Crossing the threshold once increases the short-term fluctuation, with the consequence that, although the FASTPAC algorithm offers a saving in examination time of approximately one third over the 4-2 dB algorithm, it is at the expense of increased short-term fluctuation and threshold error, which reduces the reproducibility of the test. Threshold algorithms which are faster than the 4-2 dB algorithm also exist on other perimeters, using different single step sizes, e.g. 4 dB steps or steps which vary according to the nature of the threshold (the dynamic strategy of the Octopus perimeters) but all suffer from the same disadvantages and, consequently, are not advised for use in patients where a critical diagnosis is required, e.g. glaucoma suspects.

SITA

The ideal threshold algorithm is one which can estimate the threshold with high precision, whilst simultaneously keeping the examination time to a minimum. In the mid-1990s a research group in Sweden developed a new series of threshold algorithms for the Humphrey series of perimeters which accomplish a substantial reduction in examination time relative to the standard 4-2 dB algorithm. The Swedish Interactive Threshold Algorithms, more commonly abbreviated to SITA, have effectively replaced the use of the 4-2 dB and FASTPAC algorithms. SITA employs a complex procedure to estimate the threshold. The threshold estimation procedure used in SITA requires knowledge of the frequency of seeing psychometric function at each stimulus location in the visual field, the pattern in which visual field defects occur, and how thresholds at adjacent locations in the visual field are related to each other. This "prior knowledge" enables SITA to construct mathematical models of normal and abnormal visual field behavior which are integral to the threshold estimation procedure. The abnormal model is based on threshold information gathered from patients with glaucoma, but can still be applied successfully to visual field loss resulting from other conditions. Stimuli are presented to the observer in staircases and their responses constantly update the normal and abnormal models of visual field behavior. Unlike all other threshold algorithms used in perimeters, SITA adapts the stimulus presentation speed to the reaction times of the patient, which in most cases reduces test times further.

SITA uses probability in threshold estimation. It is possible to construct a statistical distribution, or model, of probability for a given event. The shape of the probability function has a peak and width which are different, depending on the outcomes of the experiment. SITA uses Bayesian probability, which can make predictions about the nature of the threshold. Before any stimuli are presented, SITA knows the normal and abnormal behavior of the visual field. Once a threshold has been estimated, SITA adds this to the models and determines how the system should adapt in response to the information. SITA uses this probability to construct a maximum probability (MAP) estimate for the threshold. The MAP estimate is a statistical distribution of the threshold. The peak of this distribution represents the threshold estimate and the width of the distribution the accuracy of prediction of the threshold.

SITA is available in two forms; SITA Standard and SITA Fast. The difference between the two is the chosen level of accuracy for threshold estimation. Once the pre-defined level of accuracy of threshold estimation has been achieved, testing is terminated. SITA Standard has been designed to have an accuracy which is similar or better than the 4-2 dB algorithm and SITA Fast is designed to have an accuracy approaching that of FASTPAC. At the end of the examination, a brief period of post-processing occurs where vigilance criteria measured during the test are taken into account and some threshold estimates may be modified. After the post-processing period is completed, the results are made available for clinical evaluation. SITA Standard takes approximately half the time (approximately 7 minutes) to complete, than examination with the 4-2 dB algorithm. Similarly, SITA Fast takes approximately half the time of a visual field examination using the FASTPAC algorithm. As a consequence of the introduction of SITA, it is now possible to perform a full threshold static visual field examination on a patient in a time which is similar to suprathreshold examination (just over 3 minutes using SITA Fast), but which offers much greater clinical information about the visual field, thus aiding diagnosis. The SITA algorithms also incorporate novel features for monitoring patient vigilance during the visual field examination, reviewed in the following chapter.

Tendency Oriented Perimetry

SITA is the preserve of the Humphrey series of perimeters. Other perimeter manufacturers have also developed algorithms which aim to significantly reduce testing times without loss in accuracy of the threshold estimation. Tendency Oriented Perimetry (TOP) has been developed for use in the Octopus series of perimeters. Because visual field defects usually occur in patterns, e.g. a hemianopia or an arcuate defect, there is a "tendency" between thresholds in neighboring regions of the visual field. In the TOP algorithm, the estimated threshold at each stimulus location is adjusted five times, once by a direct stimulus presentation and four times from the responses to stimuli presented at neighboring locations in the visual field. The visual field is divided into four evenly inter-spaced grids, which are each examined in succession. The visual field is therefore examined in a series of adjacent matrices and the step sizes of the staircase adjusted according to a series of mathematical rules. Using the TOP strategy, examination times are comparable, if not faster, than SITA.

Spatial grid design

Regardless of the algorithm chosen to estimate thresholds in the visual field, the greater the number of stimulus presentations, the longer the duration of the visual field examination will be. The spatial grid used to evaluate the hill of vision must therefore be optimized such that the minimum number of stimulus locations yields the greatest chance or probability of detecting a visual field defect. In practice, visual field examination is primarily used for glaucoma detection and monitoring. Glaucomatous visual field loss primarily occurs in the central visual field, i.e. within 30 degrees each side of the fixation point. Two approaches exist for stimulus placement in static visual field examination. Stimuli can either be placed at regular intervals in a grid formation or placed in regions of the visual field which have the greatest likelihood of being damaged in eye disease. The probability of detecting a circular scotoma of 8.4° diameter is 100% when a square grid of 6° separation is used for stimulus presentation. Perimeters such as the Humphrey use this approach for general visual field examination. The latter approach to stimulus placement is employed in the Henson series of perimeters for suprathreshold examination (Figure 4.4).

Initially, 26 stimuli are presented in the locations in the visual field which have the greatest probability of being damaged in eye disease. If any stimuli are missed at these locations, the examination can be expanded to evaluate either 68 or 136 locations in the visual field. The 136 stimuli spatial grid is biased so that there are fewer stimuli presented in the inferior visual

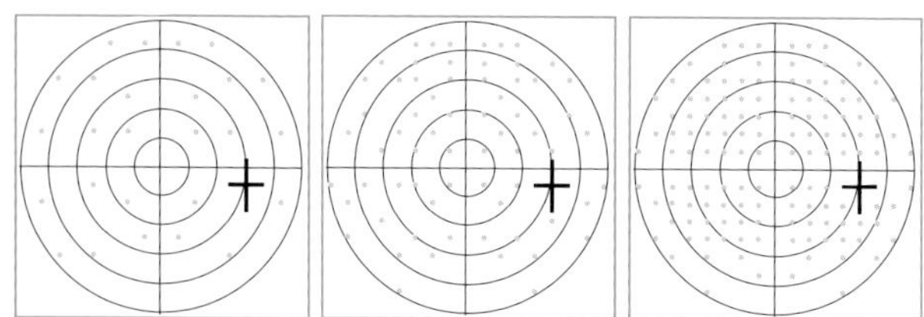

Figure 4.4 Henson perimeter sampling density

field and in the macular area. This would indicate that this grid has been optimized for the detection of glaucomatous visual field defects as they occur most commonly in the areas examined by the grid. The Octopus perimeters use regular spatial grids similar to the Humphrey and also grids designed to optimize glaucoma detection. Here the stimulus separation varies from 8 degrees in the periphery to 2 degrees in the central visual field for the detection of paracentral scotomas. The spatial grid used for stimulus presentation also depends on the eye disease being investigated. Six degree stimulus separation is entirely sufficient for the investigation of glaucoma, but is not suitable for investigation of the macular region. It should be remembered, therefore, that just because a perimeter did not detect a scotoma, it does not mean that one isn't present. Scotoma detection is determined by the size of the scotoma and the resolution of the visual field examination. The 10-2 spatial grid of the Humphrey series of perimeters uses a grid with two degree separation for investigation of the macular area. This is approximately the same separation used in Amsler grid investigation of the macular region of the visual field, but enabling full threshold examination (Figure 4.5).

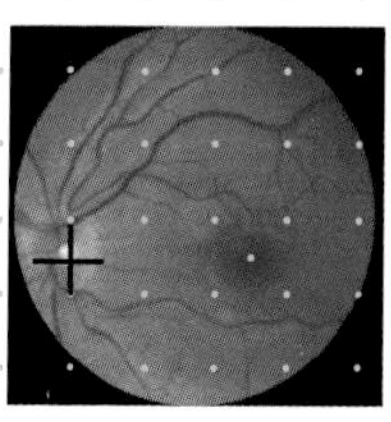

Program 30 - 2
6 degree stimulus separation

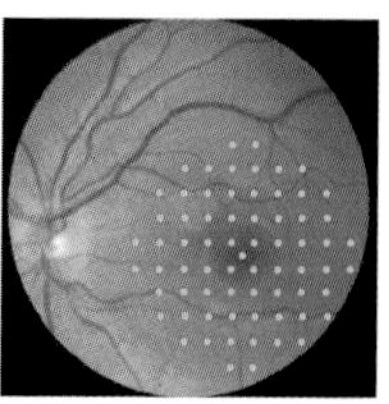

Program 10 - 2
2 degree stimulus separation

Figure 4.5 Humphrey field analyzer stimulus separation

A number of specialized spatial grids are also present on many perimeters. The most commonly used are the tests used for driving licence evaluation and are specified by the UK driving licensing authority (DVLA). Although there is some debate about the merit of these tests, they are designed to evaluate the functional vision of a driver and are usually carried out over the binocular visual field. In the Henson perimeters, the fixation point must be moved during the examination to enable placement of stimuli in the periphery of the visual field. In the Humphrey series of perimeters, the Esterman test grid is employed, but all require only a suprathreshold evaluation of the field, to identify areas of the visual field which are thought could impair driving ability.

Stimulus generation

The mode of stimulus generation differs between perimeters. In the Henson and Dicon perimeters, LED's embedded around the fixation point (in a bowl or flat surface) are used, which enable the use of multiple stimulus presentation for suprathreshold visual field examination. The use of LED's also facilitates the use of moving fixation targets. The Humphrey perimeter uses a projection system, which has the advantage that the stimulus intensity can be carefully calibrated and, if necessary, automatically adjusted using neutral density filters. Other advantages of projection of stimuli over LED's are that they enable the stimulus size and color to be altered and any spatial grid configuration can be designed. The Octopus and Oculus series of perimeters utilize a hybrid system, whereby stimuli are generated using an LED but the light output is then projected.

Summary

The major advantage of full threshold perimetry, compared to suprathreshold static examination and kinetic perimetry, is that the hill of vision is mapped with greater precision and, more importantly, the measured thresholds can be compared to a database of thresholds which are normal for an age-matched patient at a given location in the visual field, enabling statistical analysis of the visual field to be carried out, which facilitates diagnosis and monitoring of the visual field. The recent introduction of threshold algorithms such as SITA and the TOP strategy has reduced full threshold visual field examination time substantially, enabling greater patient throughput and, with increasing responsibility being given to optometric practice for monitoring glaucoma patients, the use of full threshold perimetry is set to become a more important feature of the eye examination in the future.

Further Reading

Bengtsson, B., Olsson, J., Heijl, A. and Rootzen, H. (1997). A new generation of algorithms for computerized threshold perimetry, SITA. *Acta Ophthalmol Scand.* **75**: 368–75.

Cornsweet, T.N. (1962). The staircase-method in psychophysics. *Am. J. Psychol.* **78**: 485–491.

Chauhan, B.C., Tompkins, J.D., LeBlanc, R.P. and McCormick, T.A. (1993). Characteristics of frequency-of-seeing curves in normal subjects, patients with suspected glaucoma, and patients with glaucoma. *Invest. Ophthalmol. Vis. Sci.* **34**: 3534–3540.

Flanagan, J.G., Moss, I.D., Wild, J.M., Hudson, C., Prokopich, L., Whitaker, D. and O'Neill, E.C. (1993). Evaluation of FASTPAC: a new strategy for estimation with the Humphrey Field Analyser. *Graefe's Arch. Clin. Exp. Ophthalmol.* **231**: 465–469.

Heijl, A. (1993). Perimetric point density and detection of glaucomatous visual field loss. *Acta Ophthalmologica.* **71**: 445–450.

Henson, D.B. and Anderson, R. (1989). Thresholds using single and multiple stimulus presentations. *Perimetry Update 1988/89.* Ed: Heijl, A. Amsterdam, Berkley, Milano. Kugler & Ghedini Publications, 191–196.

Gutteridge, I.F. (1984). A review of strategies for screening of the visual fields. *Aust. J. Optom.* **67**: 9–18.

Morales, J., Weitzman, M.L., de la Rosa, M.G. (2000). Comparision between Tendency-Oriented-Perimetry (TOP) and octopus threshold perimetry. *Ophthalmology* **107**: 137–142.

5
Clinical assessment of fields

Visual field examination is an easy procedure, particularly with highly automated perimeters, but the examiner should be aware of and monitor a number of factors when carrying out the test.

Setting up the patient

The patient must be set up comfortably and correctly aligned with the perimeter, in order that the visual examination is carried out efficiently. Postural discomfort can influence patient vigilance and, therefore, visual field outcome. Most perimeters incorporate an adjustable chin rest and headrest in their design. In many perimeters, the chin and head rest have been designed for both left and right eye alignment. In such rests, to examine the right eye, the chin and head must be placed on the left side of the rest and vice-versa. The chin should be firmly resting on the rest so that the head position can be altered before and during the examination, ensuring accurate placement of the light stimuli. The head must also be placed against the headrest, in order to prevent an artifact altitudinal defect forming as a result of the patient not being able to see stimuli presented in the superior visual field. The chin and head position should be checked periodically during the visual field examination to ensure the correct position has not altered.

Before asking the patient to place their chin and head against the rest, an occluding eye patch must be placed over the eye not being examined. The patient should be instructed to keep both eyes open, as some patients tend to close the occluded eye, which over time is both uncomfortable and can influence the lid position in the open eye. Patients should also be encouraged not to inhibit blinking during the test to avoid drying of the corneal surface. When using felt eye patches, the elastic should be checked to ensure that there is no tension above the eye being examined, which can affect the position of the upper eyelid. If using rigid eye patches held in place over the head by a spring, a folded tissue can be placed between the eye and the patch. If the visual field examination is to be carried out using the patient's own spectacles, consideration should be given to the size of the

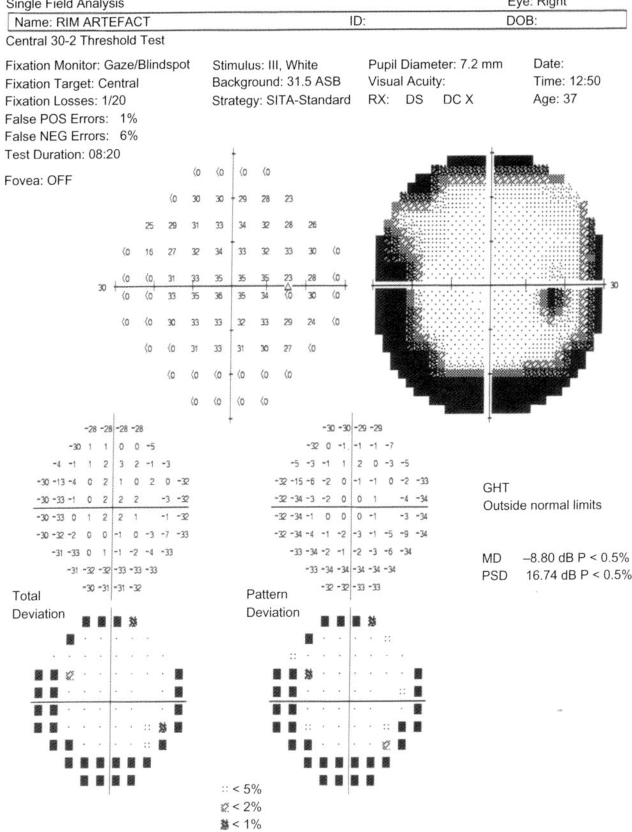

Figure 5.1 Lens rim artefact (note overall threshold value is lower than expected, giving a total deviation error)

lens aperture, as the rims of the frame could cause the formation of an artifact peripheral scotoma (Figure 5.1).

In elderly patients, superior lid ptosis may be present. Visual field examination in such patients can yield a superior visual field defect, due to the eye lid position encroaching over the

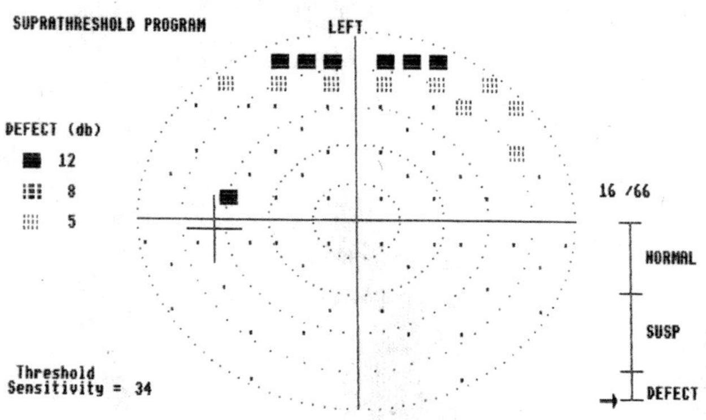

Figure 5.2 Lid scotoma. (Reproduced from Doshi and Harvey, *Investigative Techniques and Ocular Examination* (2003, Butterworth-Heinemann) with permission)

pupil (Figure 5.2). If necessary, the upper eyelid can be taped up sufficiently to prevent artifact superior visual field defects, whilst allowing the patient to maintain comfortable blinking.

Before asking the patient to place their chin on the rest, ensure that the head and chin rest are clean and sterile. If single stimulus suprathreshold or full threshold static visual field examination are to be carried out, the patient should be issued with the response button and shown its use. Any refractive correction lenses should be incorporated into the perimeter before the patient is presented to the chin and head rest. After the patient has placed their chin and head on the rest, the examiner should ensure that the outer canthus is in line with the horizontal canthus mark, which is on the side of the rest. This will ensure that there is adequate vertical movement range in the chin rest during the examination. Some perimeters additionally possess a control for lateral movement of the head to aid positioning. In order to gain accurate placement of the light stimuli, many perimeters contain a camera situated behind the fixation target. The image of the patient's eye is viewed on the perimeter control display. The center of the pupil should be positioned in the center of the cross target present on the video image. The advantage of video monitoring of the patient is that it enables the examiner to ensure that accurate fixation is taking place during the entire examination and, if necessary, correctional movements of the rest can be made.

The Goldmann perimeter, used for kinetic visual field examination, incorporates a telescope at the fixation point so that the examiner can view the patient's eye. The absence of a video or telescope monitoring system is a serious deficiency of many commonly used perimeters, as good fixation cannot be guaranteed when interpreting the results. When the examiner is satisfied that the eye position of the patient is correctly aligned, the examiner should check, firstly, the body position of the patient and alter the height of the instrument as necessary to maintain comfort and, secondly, check the head position from above the patient to ensure that the head is parallel with the horizontal dimension of the perimeter.

Refractive correction

When carrying out any visual field examination, it is imperative that the patient is corrected for refractive error appropriate for the viewing distance of the perimeter. The influence of optical defocus is to degrade the light stimulus. When no defocus is present, the detection task (the circular spot of light) is composed principally of high spatial frequencies. Optical defocus both reduces the luminance of the stimulus on the retina and increases the area of the stimulus, circularly in spherical defocus and elliptically in the case of cylindrical defocus. Under conditions of defocus, the detection task is altered to one composed mainly of low spatial frequencies. The reduced contrast of the stimulus thus influences the threshold and light sensitivity is progressively reduced as the degree of defocus increases (Figure 5.3).

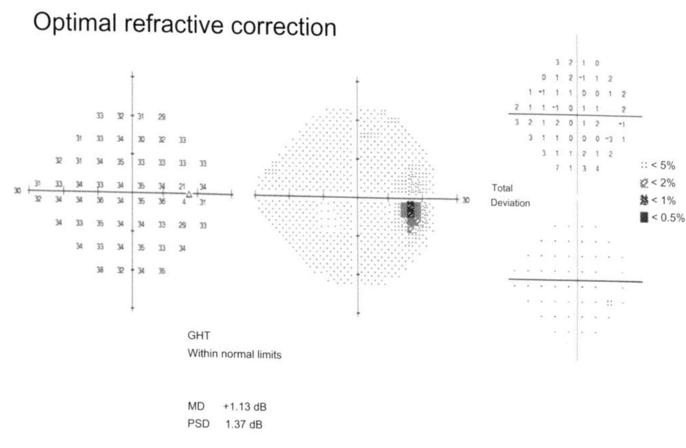

4 D of spherical defocus yields a -6.15 dB depression in sensitivity

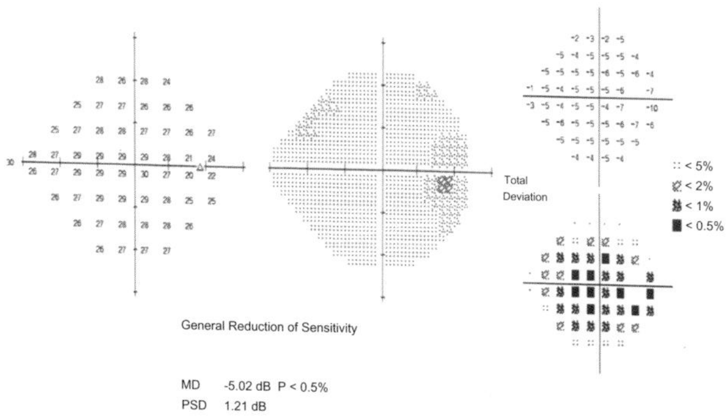

Figure 5.3 Threshold reduction resulting from a fogging lens

The increased area of the stimulus could, conceivably, result in shallow scotomas of small diameter being missed as the stimulus falls on areas of normal retinal function, masking an abnormal retinal response. In suprathreshold static examination, the testing light intensity is between 4 and 6 dB brighter than the patient's normal threshold. Therefore, it would be expected that the stimulus degradation from a small degree of optical defocus would not influence the results of the visual field examination to a large degree. However, in full threshold static visual field examination, a small degree of optical defocus would markedly influence the measured sensitivity such that statistical analysis after examination would induce a false defect. Full refractive correction must therefore be employed.

Using the mean sphere will result in significant cylindrical defocus being induced when astigmatism is greater than 1 D. Therefore, all cylinders greater than 1 D should be incorporated into the correction. Presbyopic corrections should be incorporated, suitable for the viewing distance from the rest to the fixation target; usually 25 cm or 33 cm, depending on the perimeter. Some perimeters, namely the Octopus 300 series and Oculus perimeters, incorporate an objective lens in their design, so that the light stimuli are projected to infinity. In these perimeters, the distance correction is required for patients.

The use of bifocal lenses should be avoided for two reasons; the optical defocus induced by the distance portion, and the prismatic jump induced by the segment, resulting in blind spots and displacement of stimuli. Varifocal lenses induce spherical defocus from a distance and intermediate portions and significant cylindrical defocus in the inferior peripheral portions of the lens. Consequently, only single vision lenses are suitable for perimetry.

Full aperture lenses must be used, in order that peripheral ring scotomas are not induced by the lens rim. Some perimeters provide specific head mountings for the patient to wear, incorporating corrective lenses, whilst others provide a lens mount for the addition of two lenses (usually a sphere and a cylinder). Once the patient is comfortably aligned on the perimeter rest, the vertex distance between the lens and the eye should be checked so that the lens is placed as close to the eye as possible, without obstructing lid movement. This will ensure maximum field of view during the examination and avoid the formation of an artifact rim defect.

Preparing the patient for visual field examination

Before commencing the visual field examination, adequate instruction must be given to the patient. The patient should be instructed to view the fixation target and not to look away from it at any point during the test. They should be told that periodically a light (or a number of lights in multiple stimulus suprathreshold examination) will appear somewhere in the edge of their vision. If they think they see a light they must press the response button. In multiple stimulus presentation the patient must either tell the examiner the number of lights they saw or press the response button a number of times equal to the number of lights seen. The patient should be told that there is not always a light present and they can vary in brightness from very bright to very dim. It is important to emphasize to the patient that they must watch the fixation target at all times. The default fixation target is usually a light different in color to the presentation stimuli.

In cases where the patient is known to have a central scotoma, e.g. in macular degeneration, the patient will not be able to fixate the default target. Many perimeters offer alternative fixation targets, either a cross, or four dots of light in the pattern of a cross. In these cases, good fixation can be obtained by instructing the patient to fixate the projected center of the cross.

Many perimeters incorporate a demonstration mode, whereby the patient can begin the examination, but stimulus presentation is not recorded by the perimeter. Once the examiner is satisfied the patient is carrying out the visual field examination correctly, the demonstration mode can be terminated and the visual field examination automatically begins. This gives the examiner the opportunity to reinstruct the patient if necessary. It should be remembered here that visual field examination does require a degree of concentration by the patient and it is not always possible to carry out visual field examination where there is poor patient compliance. In general, however, with accurate instruction, the vast majority of patients are able to satisfactorily complete a visual field examination.

Pupil size should not be overlooked when carrying out visual field examination, particularly where the patient is undergoing visual field monitoring. It is important to separate true improvement or worsening of the visual field outcome from alterations in pupil size, inducing change in the visual field. Pupil size determines retinal illumination, and consequently can influence visual field sensitivity. Where the pupil size has decreased significantly, relative to the previous examination, deterioration in visual field sensitivity, resulting in a worsening of the visual field outcome, would be expected. Conversely, improvement of the visual field would be expected where the pupil size has increased over successive examinations. For patients undergoing treatment for primary open-angle glaucoma, changes in pharmacological treatment regime can induce change in the visual field via change in pupil size. Such an example would be a patient who had been treated with pilocarpine, whose medication had been changed to a pharmacological agent which does not constrict the pupil. Similarly, pharmacologically induced pupil dilation for diagnostic purposes may have occurred before commencement of visual field examination. Pupil size and shape can alter significantly after ocular surgery such as cataract extraction. It is, therefore, useful to measure and record the patient's pupil size under the illumination of the visual field examination. Some perimeters which use video monitoring systems are able to measure pupil diameter automatically.

Patient monitoring during visual field examination

During the visual field examination, the examiner must constantly monitor the progress of the patient, by periodically checking and correcting the patient's head position. If necessary, the visual field examination can be paused and, with some perimeters, the patient may interrupt the examination themselves by keeping the response button depressed. During multiple stimulus examination, the patient may indicate to the examiner that they were unable to detect the correct number of stimulus presentations. This may be due to the presence of a visual field defect, but could also be due to poor concentration. It is a prudent procedure to go back to missed locations later in the examination and re-present the stimulus configuration. Often, shallow and isolated defects will disappear and enhance the final visual field interpretation.

During the course of a single stimulus suprathreshold or a full threshold visual field examination, a number of vigilance criteria are automatically assessed by the perimeter; namely, fixation losses and false negative and positive responses.

Fixation monitoring can be accomplished in a variety of ways. The crudest method is to physically watch the patient's eye via telescope or video monitoring. In the Heijl-Krakau method of fixation monitoring, a bright light stimulus is periodically presented 15 degrees from fixation along the horizontal meridian into the expected position of the physiological blind spot (Figure 5.4). If the patient is correctly fixating, they will not detect this stimulus and thus not press the response button. If the patient is not watching the fixation target when this stimulus is presented, the stimulus will not be within the physiological blind spot and the patient will respond to the stimulus, which is then recorded as a fixation loss. Some patients normally possess a displaced physiological blind spot. In these patients, the default placement of the stimulus used in the Heijl-Krakau method may be detected. This will readily be identifiable by the examiner, as the patient will appear to be fixating normally on the video monitor, but register fixation losses early in the examination. In these cases, it is possible to interrupt the visual field examination and select an option on the perimeter, instructing it to re-plot the physiological blind spot.

The Heijl-Krakau method for monitoring fixation is the commonest method used in perimetry, but it does not constantly assess fixation, requiring the examiner to watch the eye constantly during the examination (Figure 5.4).

The Humphrey and Octopus series of perimeters optical methods have been developed, by which the patient's fixation is constantly monitored during the examination. The Humphrey Field Analyser projects infra-red lights onto the cornea, enabling the perimeter to calculate the eye rotation from the distance the

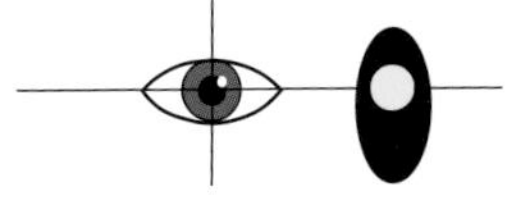

- If the patient is fixating centrally, a stimulus presented within the blind spot should not be seen.
- If the stimulus presented within the blind spot is seen, it must be because the patient is no longer fixating the central target.

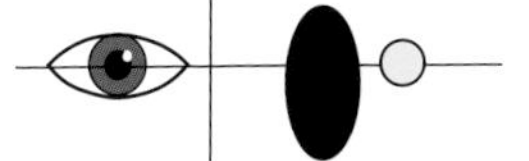

The visual field is classified as unreliable if fixation losses exceed 20%

Figure 5.4 Heijl-Krakau method of fixation monitoring

corneal reflex moves from a baseline measurement taken before the visual field examination commences. Either the examiner can correct eye movement or, in some models, the perimeter will self correct the head position during the examination (head tracking). This method of fixation monitoring is called gaze tracking and the constant real time monitoring of eye position results in the generation of a gaze graph at the end of the examination (Figure 5.5).

Upward spikes on the gaze graph indicate eye movements, whilst downward spikes indicate blinking during stimulus presentation. The examiner can then subjectively decide if fixation has been good or bad during the examination, which in turn gives an indication of how reliable the visual field outcome is. In the Octopus perimeters, the position of the pupil is measured in relation to a fixed position in the video monitoring system. The test is automatically interrupted if fixation is lost during the examination and resumes when the patient returns to the fixation target. If the patient blinks during stimulus presentation, the stimulus is represented at a later stage in the examination. Visual field outcomes are classed as unreliable when the percentage of fixation losses measured using the Heijl-Krakau method are greater than 20% of the times fixation was assessed during the examination.

Patient vigilance is also assessed periodically during the test by means of false negative and false positive catch trials. In a false

Gaze tracking (Humphrey Field Analyser 700 series)
The distance between a corneal light reflex and the center of the pupil is measured
Rotations in the eye can be distinguished from movements of the whole head
Upward deviations on the gaze graph indicate deviations due to eye movement
Downward deviation indicate that the patient blinked when a stimulus was present

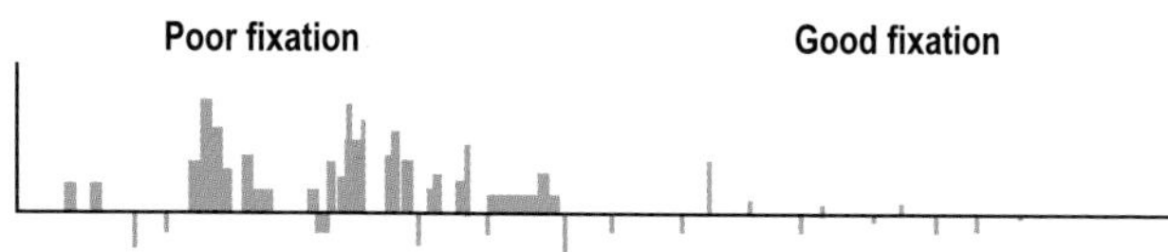

Figure 5.5 Gaze tracking

negative catch trial, a stimulus is presented at a stimulus location where threshold has already been estimated, but several decibels brighter than the threshold estimation. The patient should easily be able to detect this stimulus and respond. Should they fail to respond to the stimulus (due to inattention), a false negative response is recorded. In a false positive catch trial, the patient responds to a non-existent stimulus presentation. Many perimeters produce an audible sound which pre-conditions the patient to an imminent stimulus presentation. In a false positive catch trial, the sound is produced, but no stimulus is presented. Should the patient press the response button, a false positive catch trial is recorded. In SITA, false positives are recorded by measuring the response time of the patient. A response window of a few hundred milliseconds is allowed after the presentation of the stimulus. Should the patient press the response button outside the allowable time window, a false positive is registered. At the end of the visual field examination, the vigilance criteria are printed so that the examiner can assess the reliability of the results. In SITA, false negative and positive responses are incorporated into the visual field model and thresholds are adjusted before presentation of the final visual field result. Visual field outcomes are classed as unreliable when the percentage of false negative or positive responses exceeds 33% of the number of catch trials. A high number of false negatives during a visual examination manifest as small isolated defects and can lead to overestimation of diffuse and focal visual field loss. Conversely, a high number of false positives manifest as supra-normal sensitivity at isolated locations in the visual field and can lead to underestimation of diffuse and focal visual field loss.

In visual field examinations of long duration, e.g. a full threshold or an Esterman suprathreshold examination, the patient may become fatigued, which can profoundly influence the visual field outcome. Patient fatigue commonly begins approximately three minutes into a visual field examination. As full threshold visual field examination begins from seed points located in the central visual field, stimulus locations in the peripheral visual field have a tendency to be tested in the latter part of the examination. Consequently, in the presence of a significant fatigue effect, visual field depression may occur which is greater in the mid-peripheral and peripheral visual field. The classic presentation of the fatigue effect on visual field outcome is the clover leaf pattern (Figure 5.6), which is a result of the pattern of stimulus presentation, although fatigue can also manifest as a ring like depression in the visual field.

The causes of fatigue are not fully understood. During the course of a visual field examination, eye movements are suppressed as the patient is encouraged to maintain fixation on a central target. The uniform background against which the stimuli are presented has almost zero spatial frequency and, consequently, induces a fading effect superimposed onto the background, impairing visibility of the stimulus. This effect is termed Troxler fading or Ganzfeld blankout and is thought to be due to the influence of binocular rivalry from the occluded eye. This fading effect, which is thought to be cortical in origin, can be reduced by encouraging fixation to move during the visual field examination. Dicon perimeters periodically move the fixation target during the examination. This approach encourages saccadic eye movement, but in doing so may cause fixation instability, as the eye makes small correctional saccades after the initial pursuit movement. Psychological factors may also play a role in the fatigue effect. Visual field examination may be considered as a

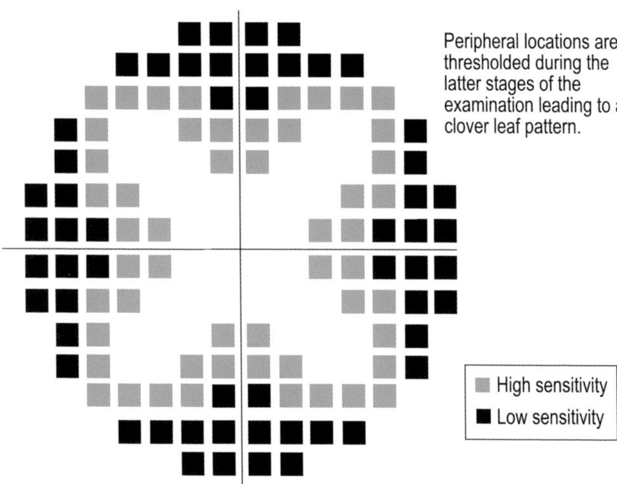

Peripheral locations are thresholded during the latter stages of the examination leading to a clover leaf pattern.
High sensitivity
Low sensitivity

Figure 5.6 Clover leaf pattern

vigilance task, since it requires a simple motor response to a randomly presented stimulus against a uniform background. The reduction in sensitivity which occurs during perimetry may result from habituation of the arousal response and increase alpha rhythm, which is associated with sleep. It is therefore important to provide regular rest periods during long visual field examinations and to encourage the patient during the course of the examination, for instance by informing them of their progress. The fatigue effect in visual field examination can be reduced, but not completely eliminated. For this reason, the second eye examined will generally perform slightly worse than the first eye, even after a significant rest period between eyes (Figure 5.7). It is therefore important, when carrying out serial visual field examination, that the eye order remains constant. The general convention is to examine the right eye before the left.

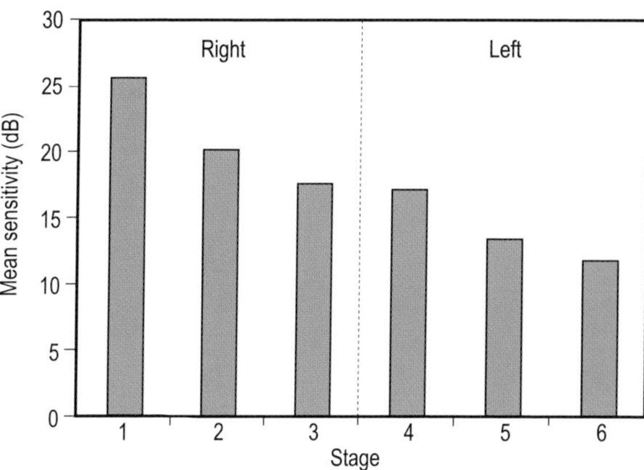

Figure 5.7 Decreasing sensitivity as visual field examination progresses (shown as stages) due to the fatigue effect. The fatigue effect "transfers" to the second eye.

Further Reading

Aman, P., Fingeret, M., Robin, A., et al. (1999). Kinetic and static fixation methods in automated threshold perimetry. *J Glaucoma* **8**: 290–296.

Atchison, D.A. (1987). Effect of defocus on visual field measurement. *Ophthal. Physiol. Opt.* **7**: 259–265.

Heijl, A. and Bengtsson, B. (1996). The effect of perimetric experience in patients with glaucoma. *Arch. Ophthalmol.* **114**: 19–22.

Heijl, A. and Krakau, C.E.T. (1975). An automatic static perimeter, design and pilot study. *Acta Ophthalmol.* **53**: 293–310

Hudson, C., Wild, J.M. and O'Neill, E.C. (1993). Fatigue effects during a single session of automated static threshold perimetry. *Invest. Ophthalmol. Vis. Sci.* **35**: 268–280.

Katz, J. and Sommer, A. (1988). Reliability indexes of automated perimetric tests. *Arch. Ophthalmol.* **106**: 1252–1254.

Lindenmuth, K.A., Skuta, G.L., Rabbani, R. and Musch, D.C. (1989). Effects of pupillary constriction on automated perimetry in normal eyes. *Ophthalmology* **96**: 1298–1301.

Lindenmuth, K.A., Skuta, G.L., Rabbani, R., Musch, D.C. and Bergstrom, T.J. (1990). Effects of pupillary dilation on automated perimetry in normal patients. *Ophthalmology* **97**: 367–370.

6
Analysis of visual field data

Analysis of kinetic perimetry

Kinetic visual field plots represent a contour map of the hill of vision, analogous to the height contours on a geographical map. The normal kinetic visual field consists of a series of isopters which are circular centrally and bound by the anatomical limits of the visual field peripherally. In the presence of focal visual field loss, the isopters deform inwards or form discrete areas of loss. Deep scotomas with steep margins are identified by closely placed isopters. Diffuse loss is more difficult to identify, as it reveals as a general constriction of the isopters. Grossly diffuse visual loss can be readily identified, but subtle diffuse loss may yield a small constriction in the isopters which is within the region of error for the placement of isopters, which is due to examiner and patient reaction times. As a result, clinical interpretation of kinetic visual fields requires a high degree of clinical experience by the examiner (Figure 6.1).

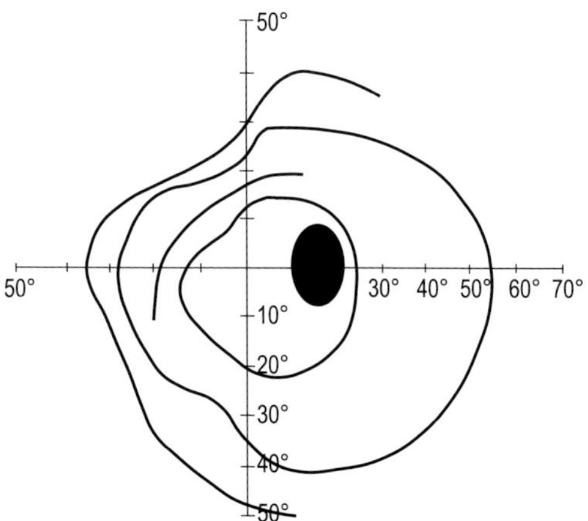

Figure 6.1 Appearance of a nasal step with kinetic perimetry

Analysis of suprathreshold static perimetry

The visual field plot from suprathreshold perimetry usually consists of a series of dots or circles, indicating the stimulus locations tested during the visual field examination, and a numerical value showing the threshold level of the patient from which the suprathreshold level was set. Dots or open circles indicate that the patient observed the suprathreshold stimulus, whereas a closed circle indicates that the patient was unable to detect the stimulus. Some perimeters quantify the visual field loss by assessing its depth using brighter stimuli. The depth of the scotoma may therefore be identified by a decibel value or a gray-scale symbol.

When single stimulus suprathreshold is carried out, the perimeter also makes measures of fixation losses, false negative and positive responses, which give the examiner an indication of the reliability of the results.

Analysis of full threshold static perimetry

The advantage of full threshold automated static perimetry over suprathreshold static perimetry is the greater information it yields about the threshold across the visual field, which enables comparison of measured data with age-matched normal data contained within the perimeter software. A number of sophisticated software packages exist to aid the practitioner in the evaluation of the final visual field outcome; each specific for a given perimeter manufacturer, the commonest being Field View (Dicon), Statpac (Humphrey) and Peri-Trend (Octopus). Basic analysis software is also contained in the Henson perimeters for full threshold evaluation. Data analysis is only possible for stimulus and grid configurations where the perimeter has age-stratified normal data. It should be remembered that, although these software packages provide diagnostic information, they should be considered as an aid to diagnosis, requiring clinical evaluation and decision-making by the practitioner. Visual field data is provided for evaluation in a variety of ways, either by a printout or electronically via a personal computer.

Numeric data

The simplest form of data presentation is a representation of threshold values in decibels arranged in the spatial locations of the test grid. Some threshold algorithms estimate the threshold twice at specific locations in the visual field. When the threshold has been determined twice it is termed a double determination. They are illustrated on the numeric printout by the two values of sensitivity (the second determination in brackets). The numeric printout permits the display of the raw data prior to statistical manipulation. High numbers represent regions of high light sensitivity in the visual field. In a normal visual field, the inferior visual field generally exhibits slightly higher sensitivity than the superior visual field. Sensitivities are greatest in the central visual field and exhibit a gradual decline towards the visual field periphery, reflecting the shape of the hill of vision. A decibel value of 0 dB indicates detection of the brightest light stimulus the perimeter is able to generate. A value of < 0 dB indicates that the patient was unable to detect the maximum stimulus luminance (differing between perimeters but typically in the order of 10,000 asb), but this does not necessarily mean that the patient has no light perception in that region of the visual field. Although the numeric printout gives the practitioner some indication of areas of defect in the visual field, the large amounts of such data do not facilitate interpretation of the visual field.

Color-scale

The color scale aims to display sensitivity values in a map form in order that it can be more readily interpreted than numeric data (Figure 6.2).

Ranges of sensitivity values are represented by different colors (dark colors indicating low sensitivity and light colors high

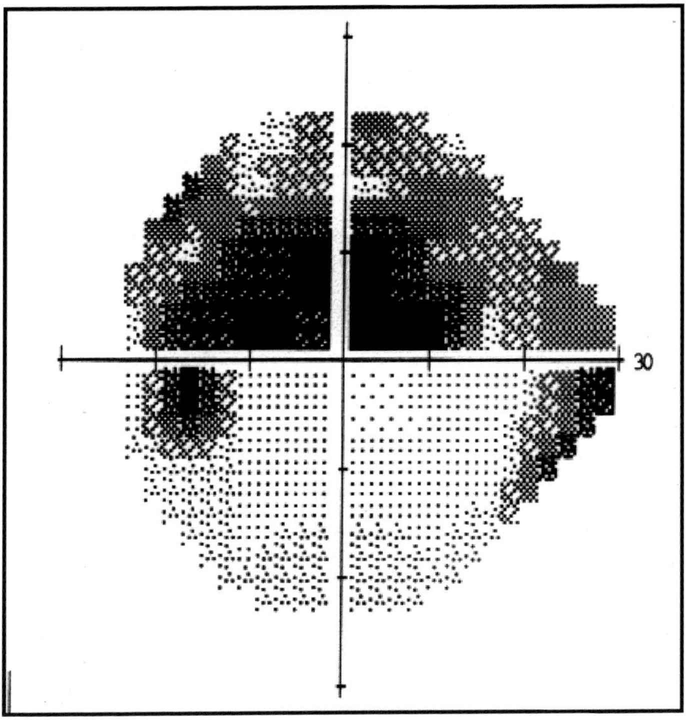

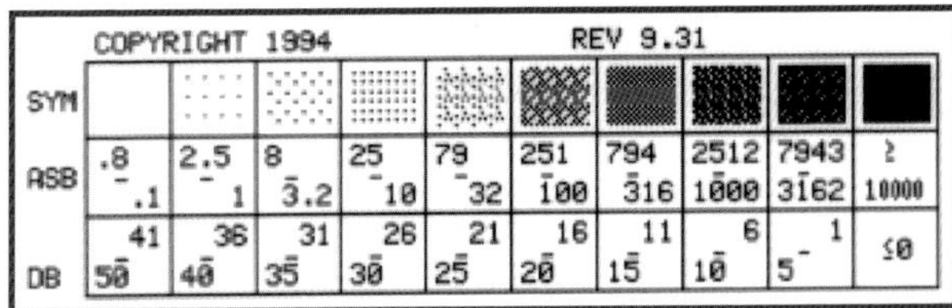

COPYRIGHT 1994 REV 9.31

SYM										
ASB	.8 - .1	2.5 - 1	8 - 3.2	25 - 10	79 - 32	251 - 100	794 - 316	2512 - 1000	7943 - 3162	≥ 10000
DB	41 - 50	36 - 40	31 - 35	26 - 30	21 - 25	16 - 20	11 - 15	6 - 10	1 - 5	≤0

Figure 6.2 Color scale map

sensitivity) or in shades of gray (black indicating low sensitivity and white high sensitivity). Sensitivity values are generally banded into 5 dB groupings, with regions between the locations tested illustrated by interpolation. The disadvantage of color scales is that a particular location in the visual field may have high sensitivity but may still be abnormal, or that a location may have depressed sensitivity relative to the surrounding locations, which is suspicious, but all locations fall within a particular decibel grading color and thus will not readily appear as a defect. A modification to the standard color scale is used in the Field-View package, in which it is possible to view the color scale as a fully rotational 3-dimensional hill of vision, in which colors indicate regions of sensitivity and the depth of scotomas is shown as changes in the relief of the hill of vision.

Probability plots

Probability plots are another form of graphical presentation of visual field data which are superior to examination of the numeric printout or color-scale maps, because they make comparisons of measured sensitivity with age-matched normal sensitivity on a point-by-point basis, yielding an outcome on the likelihood of a given location being normal or abnormal. In order to understand probability plots it is first necessary to understand the normal age related decline in sensitivity of the visual field. The normal visual field reduces in height and becomes steeper as age advances.

The normal decline in visual field sensitivity is on average approximately 0.7 dB per decade and is thought to be due to a progressive age-related loss in photoreceptors and neural cells, in addition to a general decrease in the clarity of the optical media, reducing stimulus detection via light absorption and scatter. Figure 6.3 illustrates this decline in light sensitivity with age across the normal visual field at a central and a peripheral stimulus location.

There is a normal variation in light sensitivity for a given age with greater variation present in the peripheral than the central visual field. When presented with a range of normal values, it is possible to statistically define the arithmetic mean, but more importantly define confidence intervals for a normal population. The dotted lines in figure 6.3 indicate the 95% confidence interval. Within the boundaries of these confidence intervals 95% of all normal sensitivities are contained. If a sensitivity is measured in a patient and it falls outside this range, it will be

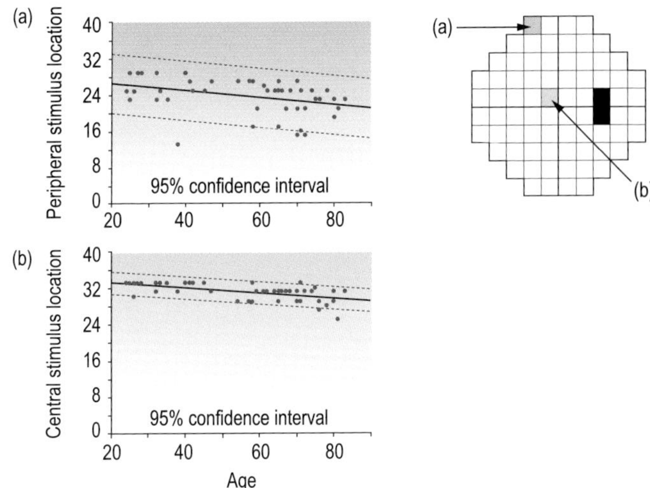

Figure 6.3 Decline in sensitivity of central and peripheral retina with age

assigned a P<5% probability level, meaning that the measured sensitivity is normal in less than 5% of the normal population (because the 95% confidence limits contain 95% of the normal value). Thus, probability plots graphically illustrate the level of statistical significance associated with a given visual field abnormality compared to the normal reference field. Visual field locations with statistically abnormal sensitivity do not necessarily mean that the measured sensitivity is abnormal, but there is a very high likelihood of being so, particularly when probability symbols appear in clusters. The reasons for the abnormal sensitivity may be due to damage to the visual pathway but could also be due to factors such as inattention during the visual field examination, which is why the practitioner must consider this information in conjunction with other visual field analyses and clinical data when making a clinical interpretation.

In visual field analysis there are two types of probability plots, one sensitive to the detection of diffuse visual loss (the total deviation plot, Figure 6.4 a and b) and the other sensitive to the detection of focal visual field loss (the pattern deviation plot, Figure 6.5 a and b).

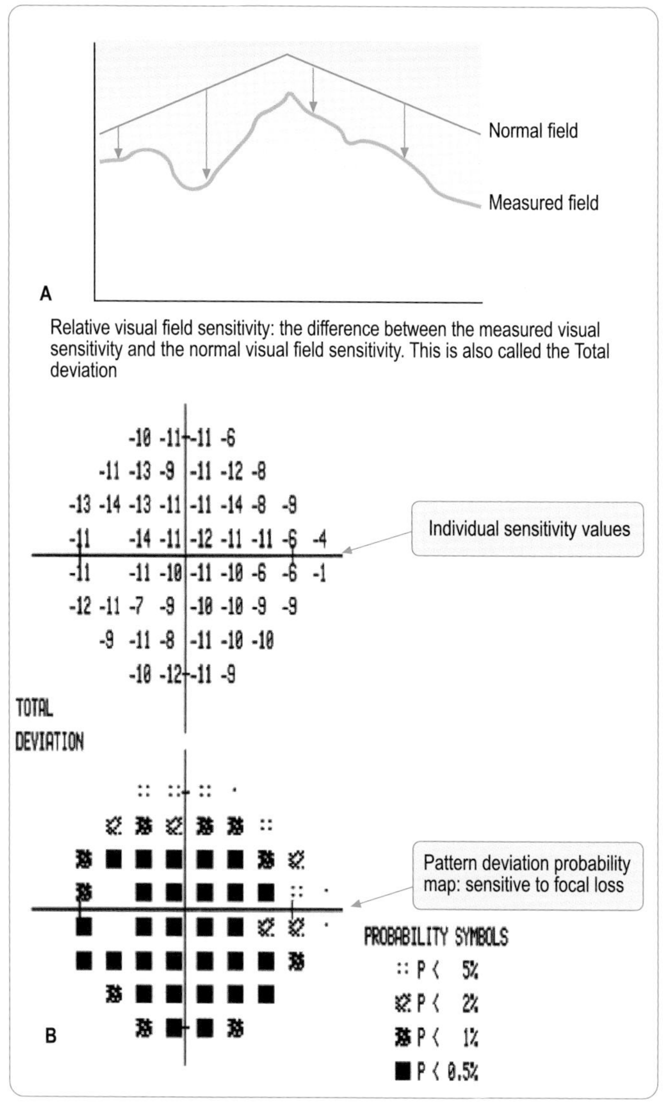
Normal field
Measured field
A
Relative visual field sensitivity: the difference between the measured visual sensitivity and the normal visual field sensitivity. This is also called the Total deviation
-10 -11 -11 -6
-11 -13 -9 -11 -12 -8
-13 -14 -13 -11 -11 -14 -8 -9
-11 -14 -11 -12 -11 -11 -6 -4
-11 -11 -10 -11 -10 -6 -6 -1
-12 -11 -7 -9 -10 -10 -9 -9
-9 -11 -8 -11 -10 -10
-10 -12 -11 -9
TOTAL
DEVIATION
Individual sensitivity values
Pattern deviation probability map: sensitive to focal loss
PROBABILITY SYMBOLS
:: P < 5%
P < 2%
P < 1%
P < 0.5%
B

Figure 6.4 Total deviation probability plot

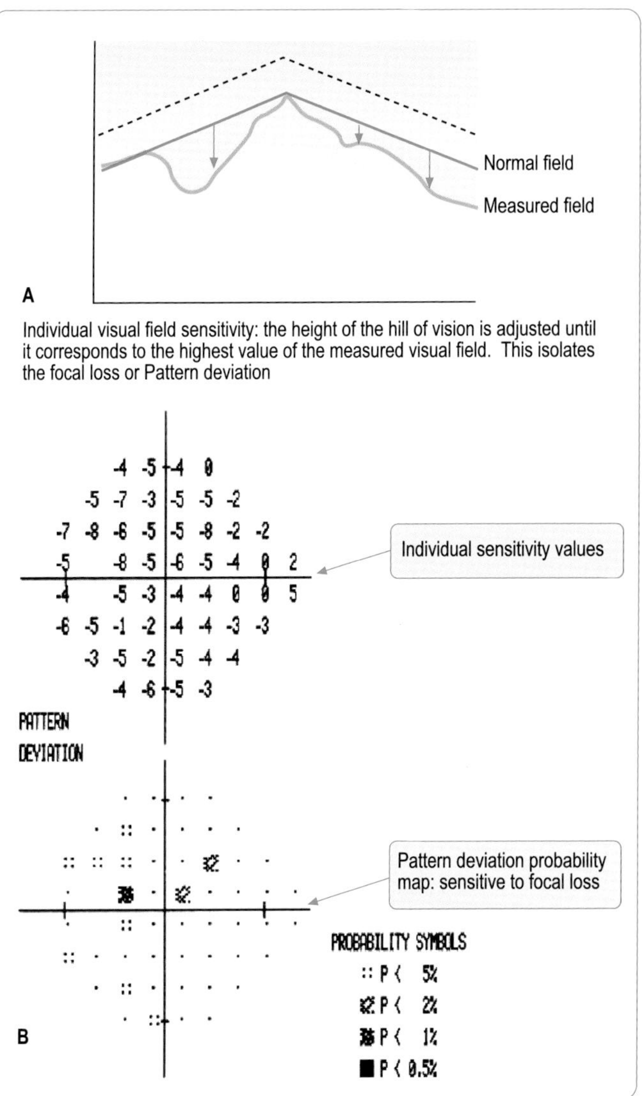
Normal field
Measured field
A
Individual visual field sensitivity: the height of the hill of vision is adjusted until it corresponds to the highest value of the measured visual field. This isolates the focal loss or Pattern deviation
-4 -5 -4 0
-5 -7 -3 -5 -5 -2
-7 -8 -6 -5 -5 -8 -2 -2
-5 -8 -5 -6 -5 -4 0 2
-4 -5 -3 -4 -4 0 0 5
-6 -5 -1 -2 -4 -4 -3 -3
-3 -5 -2 -5 -4 -4
-4 -6 -5 -3
Individual sensitivity values
PATTERN
DEVIATION
Pattern deviation probability map: sensitive to focal loss
PROBABILITY SYMBOLS
P < 5%
P < 2%
P < 1%
P < 0.5%
B

Figure 6.5 Pattern deviation probability plot

In the total deviation plot, the difference between the measured visual field sensitivity and the expected normal visual field sensitivity are plotted as a numeric map. A second plot illustrates those locations where the deviation is significantly different from the normal population, either at the P <0.5%, P <1%, P <2% or P <5% levels.

The pattern deviation probability map separates the general reduction in sensitivity, which may arise through media opacities, optical defocus or pupillary miosis (total deviation) from the localized reduction in sensitivity. In order to calculate the pattern deviation probability map, locations within 24 degrees of fixation are ranked according to the deviation in sensitivity compared to the age-matched normal population. General sensitivity is calculated from the measured value of the seventh highest deviation (85th percentile) in sensitivity. The patient in Figure 6.6 clearly shows large areas of focal loss on the pattern deviation consistent with a superior arcuate scotoma.

Over time these locations are likely to worsen, with both the level of significance and the number of locations increasing. The probability map is therefore of use when monitoring a patient over time. Caution with these plots should be applied, however, when small isolated areas of loss are found, such as in Figure 6.7.

These locations may be of significance merely because of noise generated in the data. The patient's fundus should be examined to see whether there is a pathological cause for the visual field loss. If none can be found, then the patient's visual field should be repeated at a later date. Clusters of probability symbols are of greater clinical significance than scattered isolated symbols. Only if the visual field defect is repeatable should the patient be considered for referral to a specialist.

Global visual field indices

Graphical displays such as color-scales suffer from a number of disadvantages, namely that they inadequately define diffuse visual field loss and changes between a series of visual fields. Statistical interpretation of perimetric data does not suffer from these

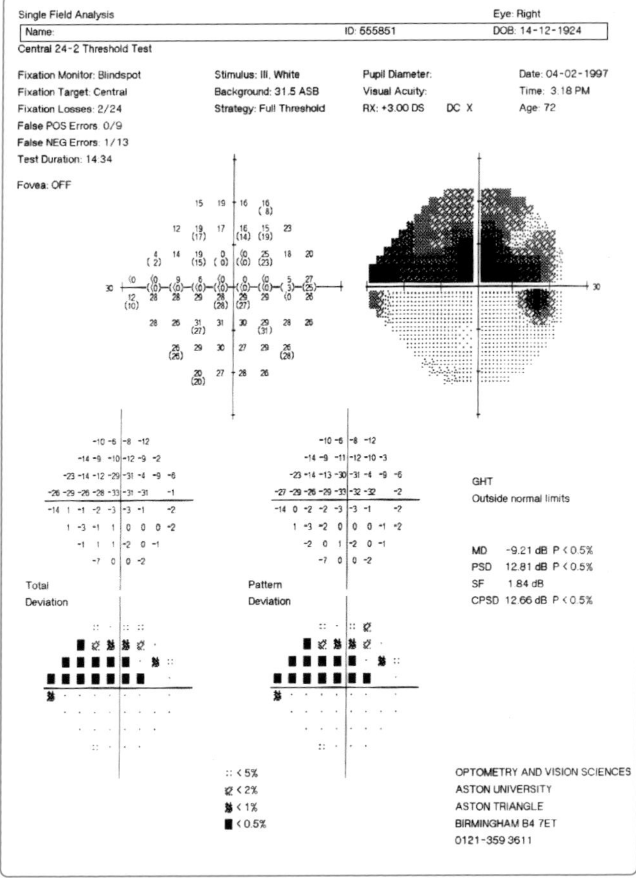

Figure 6.6 Superior arcuate scotoma

disadvantages. Global visual field indices are a useful method of data reduction, since they yield a single number which is an indication of the degree of diffuse or focal loss in the visual field. They are also of use when evaluating visual field change over time. A wide variety of visual field indices have been developed for the Octopus and Humphrey Field Analyser perimeters to summarize the data reduction at each stimulus location.

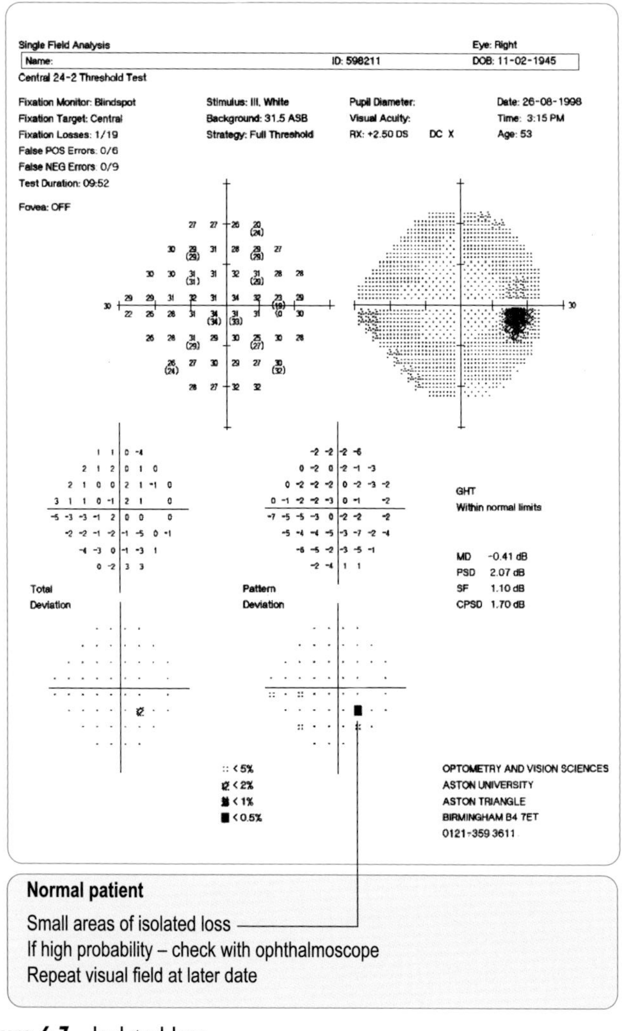

Figure 6.7 Isolated loss

Mean sensitivity

Mean sensitivity (MS) simply represents the arithmetic mean of the measured sensitivity at all stimulus locations tested in the visual field. Since there is no reference to the patient's age this index is of little use clinically.

Mean defect and mean deviation

The mean defect (MD) is the arithmetic mean of the difference between the measured values and the normal values at the different test locations. This statistic is employed in the Octopus and Henson perimeters. A positive MD represents a loss of sensitivity. The index is sensitive to diffuse visual field loss but is relatively unaffected by focal loss. Thus, in the presence of cataract, the MD will be increased.

The equivalent index used in the Humphrey Field Analyzer is mean deviation, which is also abbreviated to MD. Mean deviation is a weighted average deviation from the normal reference visual field. A negative mean deviation represents a loss in sensitivity. It is important to check whether the MD index represents mean defect or mean deviation. In the presence of a large focal loss the MD will also be increased because a large number of locations will be depressed, which influences the mean sensitivity (Figures 6.8a and b).

Loss variance (standard deviation defect) and pattern standard deviation

The loss variance (LV) statistic of the Octopus perimeter describes the non-uniformity in the height of the visual field. It is small if visual field damage is diffuse (e.g. in cataract) and is high in the presence of focal loss (e.g. in glaucoma or hemianopia) (Figures 6.8a and b). Variations in this index occur in other perimeters; in the Henson series it is called the standard

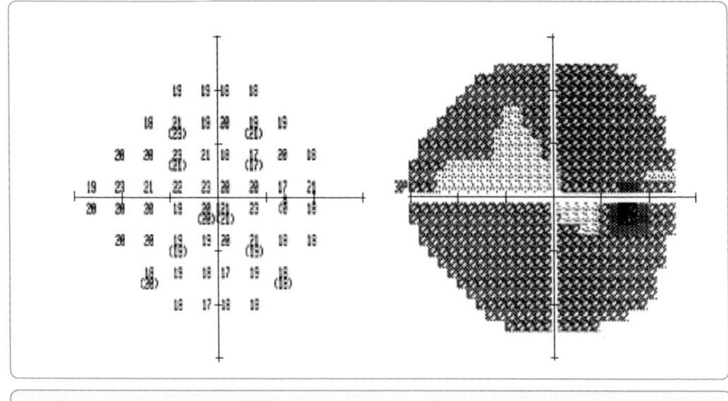

MD   -8.71 dB   P < 0.5%   Values greater than ± 2.00 dB are usually abnormal
PSD   2.15 dB
SF   0.97 dB
CPSD   1.88 dB   P < 10%

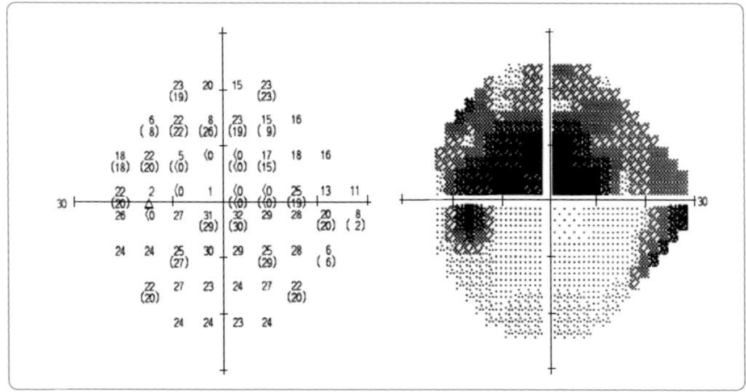

MD   -11.01 dB   P < 0.5%   Values greater than + 2.00 dB are usually abnormal
PSD   11.85 dB   P < 0.5%
SF   2.01 dB
CPSD   11.66 dB   P < 0.5%

Figure 6.8 (a) Mean deviation in cataract; (b) Mean deviation in glaucoma

deviation defect. The pattern standard deviation (PSD) statistic of the Humphrey Field Analyser is a weighted standard deviation of the differences between the measured and normal reference visual field at each stimulus location (Figure 6.9).

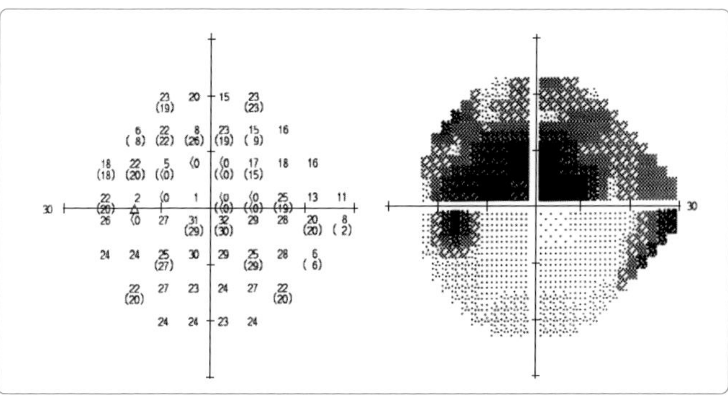

MD	-11.01 dB	P < 0.5%	
PSD	11.85 dB	P < 0.5%	Values greater than ± 2.00 dB are usually abnormal
SF	2.01 dB		
CPSD	11.66 dB	P < 0.5%	

Figure 6.9 Pattern standard deviation in glaucoma

It is analogous to loss variance and standard deviation defect. The patient in Figure 6.7 has a very small isolated area of focal loss and the PSD is unaffected. However, the patient in Figure 6.6 has a large area of focal loss reflected by the magnitude of the PSD.

Short-term fluctuation

The variability in the sensitivity which occurs when a threshold is estimated repeatedly during a single visual field examination is termed the short-term fluctuation (SF). In the Octopus perimeter it is the average of the local scatter over the entire visual field, determined from the square root of the sum of the local standard deviations averaged over the visual field. Calculation of SF in this way assumes that the variance is constant at all locations in the visual field. However, the variance is known to increase with eccentricity.

The G1 program of the Octopus perimeter estimates the SF from double determinations of threshold at each location in the

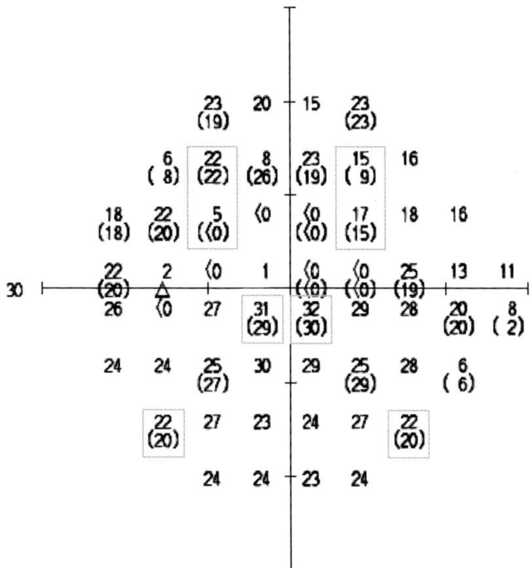

Figure 6.10 Stimulus locations used for the calculation of short-term fluctuation in the Humphrey Field Analyzer

visual field, obtained over two phases. The 30-2 and 24-2 programs of the Humphrey Field Analyser estimate SF from double determinations of threshold, obtained from ten locations within 21° eccentricity (Figure 6.10). The SF is greater around the borders of a scotoma, since small movements in fixation may result in the first and second threshold determination falling within and outside a scotoma, respectively. Therefore, a high SF may be indicative of a pathological visual field.

Corrected loss variance and corrected pattern standard deviation

Corrected loss variance (CLV), corrected standard deviation defect and corrected pattern standard deviation (CPSD) are represented as the LV, standard deviation defect and PSD corrected for the SF. They are, therefore, indices which are sensitive to focal loss and may separate real deviations from those deviations which are due to variability. Since SITA adjusts thresholds for variability, the SF and CPSD indices do not need to be calculated.

The Glaucoma Hemifield Test

The Glaucoma Hemifield Test (GHT) was introduced in the Humphrey Field Analyzer with the aim of deciding whether visual field loss was compatible with a diagnosis of glaucoma. Ten anatomical sectors in the visual field are superimposed on the Program 30-2 test grid, selected according to the normal arrangement of retinal nerve fibers. Five sectors in the upper hemifield mirror five sectors in the inferior field. Probability scores are calculated for each location within the ten sectors, according to the pattern deviation probability map. Within each sector, the sum of the probability scores is calculated and the difference compared to the mirror image sector. A visual field is classed as "outside normal limits" if the difference in any of the five corresponding pairs of sectors falls outside the 0.5% or 99.5% confidence limits for that pair of sectors. Visual fields are classified as "borderline" if any sector-pair difference exceeds the 3% confidence limit. If the general height of the field is below the 0.5% limit, the GHT evaluates the field as a "general reduction in sensitivity". A classification of "abnormally high sensitivity" is associated with a high level of false-positive responses. The general height test is not performed if the visual field has already been classified as "outside normal limits". A sensitivity and specificity of 80.8% and 81.4% respectively has been reported for the GHT. The GHT also gives an indication of patient reliability, flagging "low patient reliability" should fixation losses, false negative and positive responses lie outside the limits discussed earlier (Figure 6.11).

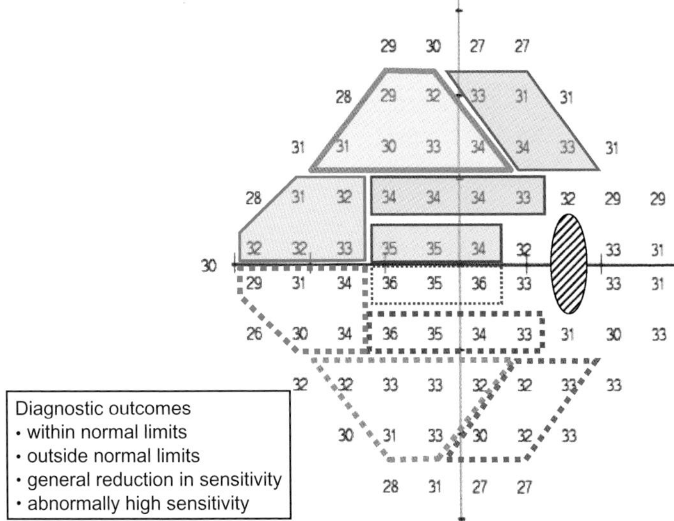

Figure 6.11 Optic nerve fiber sectors (solid lines) and their mirror images (dotted lines) used for comparison in the Glaucoma Hemifield Test of the Humphrey Field Analyzer

Bebié curve

The Bebié curve is a cumulative distribution of the defect depth at each location and is designed to separate normal visual fields from those with early diffuse loss (Figure 6.12).

The defect depth is sorted into ascending order of severity and plotted as a function of rank. A shaded zone is employed to aid interpretation of the resultant curve. The enclosed region corresponds to the 5th and 95th percentiles. A normal visual field yields a curve above or closely following the 95th percentile line. A curve falling below (i.e. outside) the 95th percentile line indicates visual field loss. A visual field with purely diffuse loss will mimic the shape of the curve associated with normality, but at a greater overall defect depth. Focal loss is indicated by a steepening of the curve. A clear boundary does not separate diffuse from focal loss on the curve. Furthermore, the Bebié

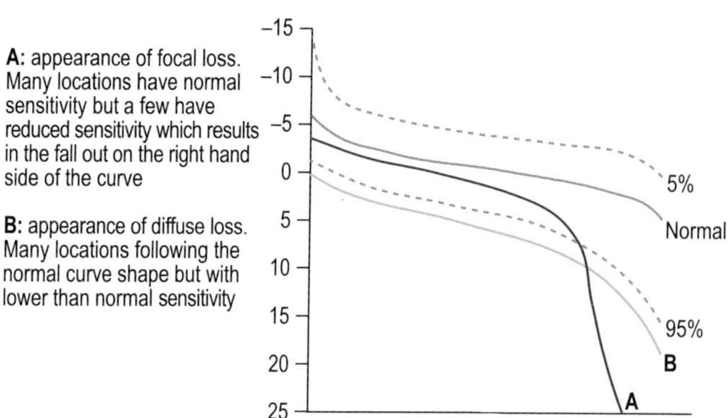

pattern of normal sensitivities
A: appearance of focal loss. Many locations have normal sensitivity but a few have reduced sensitivity which results in the fall out on the right hand side of the curve
B: appearance of diffuse loss. Many locations following the normal curve shape but with lower than normal sensitivity
−15
−10
−5
0
5
10
15
20
25
5%
Normal
95%
B
A

Figure 6.12 The Bebié curve

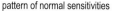

curve does not yield information about the spatial characteristics of the visual field loss and may not detect central visual field depressions in early glaucoma.

Statistical interpretation of the visual field aids the practitioner when deciding whether or not visual field loss is present and, in the case of serial examination, when determining whether or not visual field progression has occurred. However, it should be remembered that a degree of clinical judgement is also required when evaluating visual fields and the results must be used in conjunction with other clinical data when making decisions regarding patient management.

Data analysis

The imprecision in the staircase and the large number of locations where estimation of the threshold occurs create a degree of noise in the data gathering process, which must be filtered out as much as possible to enable statistical interpretation. The short-term fluctuation assists in the filtering of threshold variability and improves global measures of focal visual field loss. Other psychological factors, such as the learning effect (Figure 6.13), whereby a patient's visual field sensitivity improves

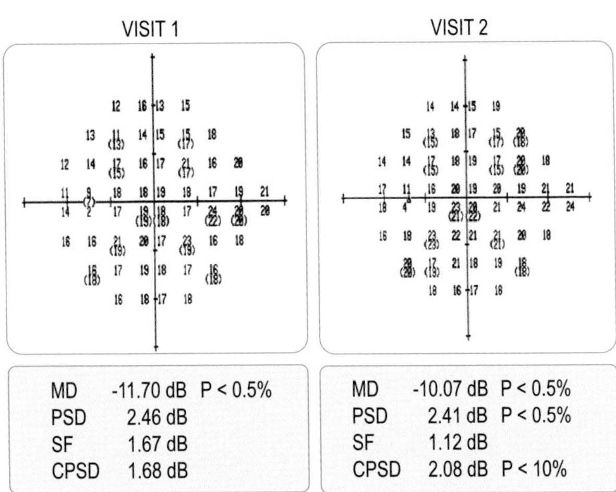

Figure 6.13 Learning effect across two consecutive visits

over successive examinations, and the fatigue effect (which reduces sensitivity during the course of an examination) also need to be considered when evaluating a visual field.

Serial visual field analysis

One of the advantages of statistical analysis is that it enables successive visual fields to be analyzed for change. In its simplest form, change can be monitored by looking for deterioration or improvement in the global visual field indices. As glaucoma progresses, the extent of focal visual field loss becomes greater and defects become deeper. This causes the PSD (or LV) and the MD indices to increase. Similarly, the significance of probability symbols increases and clusters of symbols become larger. In cataract, the MD index and total deviation probability would be expected to worsen. One of the difficulties in examining serial visual fields is the differentiation of abnormal areas from areas of noise, signified by non-repeatable test locations and excluding improvement in the visual field due to the learning effect or visual field deterioration, due to the fatigue effect. Many of the perimeter programs for statistical analysis of visual fields incorporate packages which analyze change in the visual field. The most sophisticated of these is found in the Humphrey Field Analyser, which offers several means of monitoring change. The simplest method is the analysis of the mean deviation index, which can be plotted as a function of change (linear regression). Within the perimeter database is a subset of data from a group of stable glaucoma patients. The change in MD over time can be compared with this group and illustrated graphically to show whether significant visual field progression has occurred over time. Stable glaucoma patients are expected to yield greater fluctuation with eccentricity and depth of defect. The measured points of the patient are expected to demonstrate greater change in order to be statistically significant.

Another graphical display of change are box plots, which are a modified bar graph of the threshold values. The ranked difference between the measured and expected values are calculated and ranked. The box represents the range of deviation for the middle 70% of stimulus locations, i.e. the standard deviation. The upper

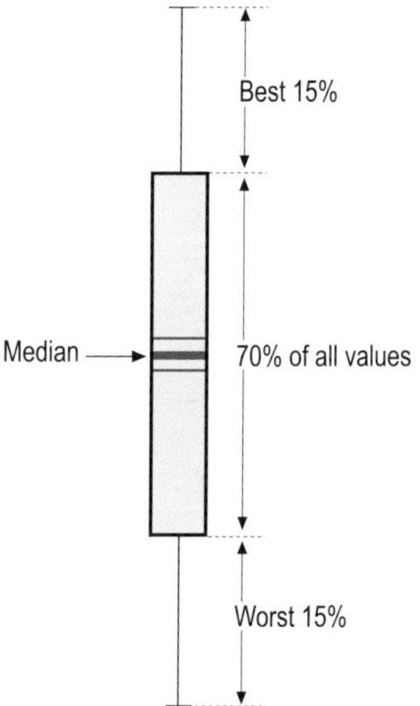

Figure 6.14 Normal box plot presentation

tail represents the range of the 15% best stimulus locations and the lower tail the range of the 15% worst stimulus locations (Figure 6.14).

Box plots for each examination are shown next to a reference normal plot. When the plot has the same shape as normal but is graphed at a lower point to the middle reference line, a depression in height of the hill of vision is indicated, i.e. diffuse visual field loss. If the bottom of the box is in the same position as normal but the tail is elongating, a deepening of focal loss is indicated. If the bottom of the box lowers, but the median remains in the same position relative to the normal, enlargement of focal loss is indicated. Finally, if the bottom of the box lowers, the top shrinks in height and the median worsens, enlargement of focal loss is suspected (Fig 6.15).

The most sophisticated analysis program on the Humphrey Visual Field Analyser is the glaucoma change probability (GCP) program (Figure 6.16).

This analysis requires a minimum of three visual fields to be carried out. In order to minimize the learning effect, two early and consecutive visual fields are combined to form an average "baseline" visual field. The analysis is displayed as a grayscale and a

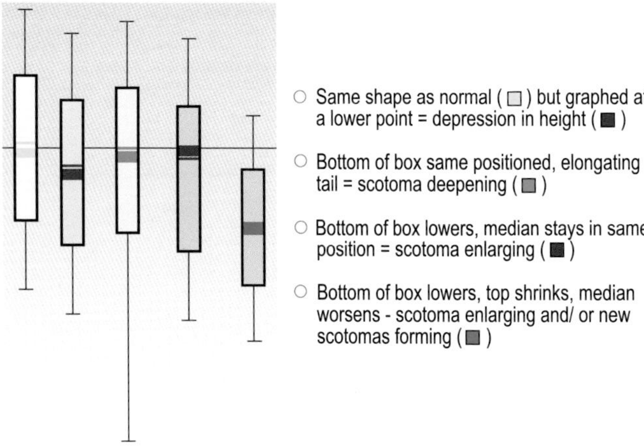

Same shape as normal ( ) but graphed at a lower point = depression in height ( )
Bottom of box same positioned, elongating tail = scotoma deepening ( )
Bottom of box lowers, median stays in same position = scotoma enlarging ( )
Bottom of box lowers, top shrinks, median worsens - scotoma enlarging and/ or new scotomas forming ( )

Figure 6.15 Diagnostic outcomes of the box plot

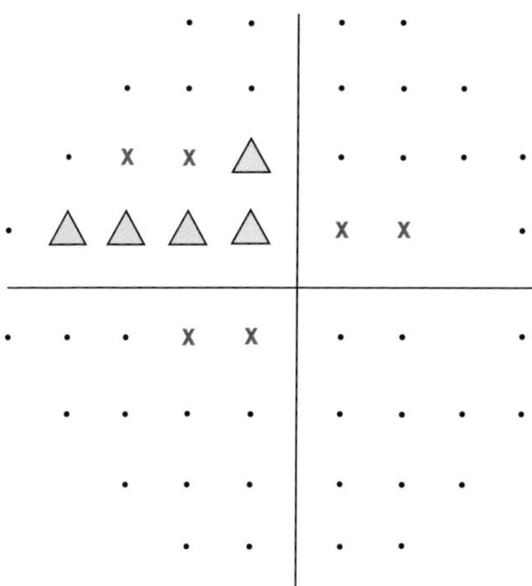

• Normal sensitivity

▲ Significantly decreased sensitivity compared to baseleine

△ Significantly increased sensitivity compared to baseline

x If MD > — 15 dB STATPAC cannot determine significant change

Figure 6.16 Glaucoma change probability analysis

second total deviation plot, which shows any stimulus location which has significantly changed from the baseline. A third plot shows the glaucoma change probability. Normal locations are shown as a dot. Locations which have decreased sensitivity compared to the baseline are shown as closed triangles and those which yield improved sensitivity relative to the baseline are shown as open triangles. If the MD is greater than –15 dB, the analysis program cannot determine the significance of the change and such locations are illustrated with a cross. It is possible that a stable glaucomatous visual field can simultaneously show a few improved and deteriorated locations. True deterioration can only be established if the location is repeatable at the next examination. GCP does not account for any change in the visual field which is due to conditions other than glaucoma, such as cataract or pupil size change due to changes in glaucoma therapy.

The deficiencies of GCP have, to a large extent, been overcome by the recent upgrade of the progression analysis software; glaucoma change analysis, which incorporates the advances of SITA and the results of a multi-center research study into glaucoma visual field progression into the software. The new change analysis software highlights, with an open triangle, stimulus locations which show progression at the 95% confidence level; a half open triangle represents locations where progression has occurred and is repeatable after two examinations and closed triangles represent where progression is repeatable after three examinations. The new analysis also corrects for changes in ocular media density, thus enabling the separation of change due to diffuse loss and that of glaucoma. Although change analysis programs are becoming more sophisticated all the time, it should be remembered that they are only a guide to diagnosis. The final diagnosis should always rest with the clinician.

Further Reading

Åsman, P. and Heijl, A. (1992). Glaucoma Hemifield Test. Automated visual field evaluation. *Arch. Ophthalmol.* **110**: 812–819.

Bebié, H., Flammer, J. and Bebié, T. (1989). The cumulative defect curve: separation of local and diffuse components of visual field damage. *Graefe's Arch. Clin. Exp. Ophthalmol.* **227**: 9–12.

Flammer, J. (1986). The concept of visual field indices. *Graefe's Arch. Clin. Exp. Ophthalmol.* **224**: 389–392.

Flammer, J., Drance, S.M. and Zulauf, M. (1984). Differential light threshold. Short- and long-term fluctuation in patients with glaucoma, normal controls, and patients with suspected glaucoma. *Arch. Ophthalmol.* **102**: 704–706.

Greve, E.L. (1973). Single and multiple stimulus static perimetry in glaucoma; the two phases of perimetry. *Doc. Ophthalmol.* **36**: 1–355.

Heijl, A., Lindgren, G. and Olsson, J. (1987). A package for the statistical analysis of visual fields. *Documenta Ophthalmologica Proceedings Series 49*. Proceedings of the Seventh International Visual Field Symposium. Eds: Greve, E.L. and Heijl, A. Dordrecht. Martinus Nijhoff / Dr. W. Junk Publishers, pp. 593–600.

Heijl, A., Lindgren, G., Lindgren, A., Olsson, J., Åsman, P., Myers, S. and Patella, M. (1991). Extended empirical statistical package for evaluation of single and multiple fields in glaucoma: Statpac 2. *Perimetry Update 1990/91*. Proceedings of the IXth International Perimetric Society Meeting. Eds: Mills, R.P. and Heijl, A. Amsterdam, New York and Milano. Kugler & Ghedini, pp. 303–315.

Johnson, C.A. and Keltner, J.L. (1987). Optimal rates of movement for kinetic perimetry. *Arch. Ophthalmol.* **105**: 73–75.

Katz, J. (2000). A comparison of the pattern- and the total deviation-based glaucoma probability programs. *Invest Ophthalmol Vis Sci.* **41**: 1012–1016.

Morgan, R.K., Feuer, W.J. and Anderson, D.R. (1991). Statpac 2 glaucoma change probability. *Arch. Ophthalmol.* **109**: 1690–1692.

Weber, J. and Geiger, R. (1989). Grey scale display of perimetric results – the influence of different interpolation procedures. In: *Perimetry Update 1988/89*. Proceedings of the VIIth International Perimetric Society. Ed: Heijl, A. Amsterdam, Berkeley and Milano. Kugler & Ghedini, pp. 447–454.

7 Advanced techniques for the investigation of the visual field

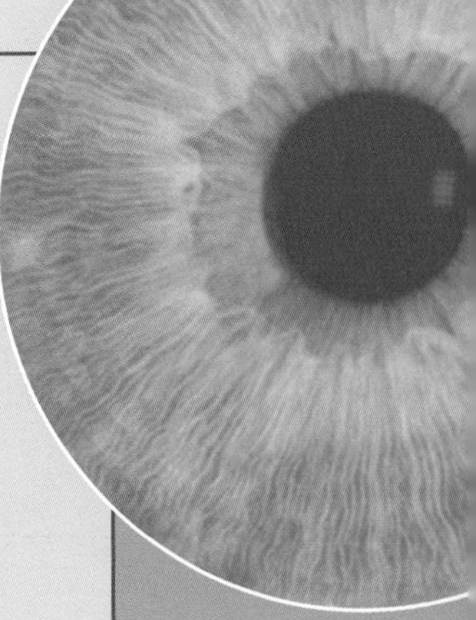

Visual field examination using automated static perimetry has become the standard clinical tool for the diagnosis and monitoring of glaucoma in optometric practice and ophthalmology. Glaucoma is defined as an optic neuropathy causing characteristic optic nerve head cupping and visual field loss. Although automated static perimetry is the most sensitive tool used for the diagnosis and monitoring of glaucoma in clinical practice, it does not detect glaucoma until the disease process is well advanced. There are a number of other disease processes where significant structural changes occur to the retina before they can be detected with standard visual field investigation. Numerous research groups around the world have attempted to develop new and commercial methods of visual field examination which aim to detect these disease processes in their earliest stages (centering primarily on glaucoma), with the hope that earlier treatment of the disease may arrest damage to the visual pathway.

In glaucoma, histological studies on post-mortem eyes have shown that up to 50% of optic nerve head fibers are lost before a visual field defect manifests with standard automated static perimetry. The current drug and surgical therapies used for the treatment of glaucoma significantly slow the rate of progression of the disease, but do not cure the condition. During the 1980's a number of histological studies concluded that larger optic nerve fibers are damaged earliest in the glaucomatous disease process. This led to the selective damage hypothesis, which states that larger retinal nerve fibers are damaged earliest in glaucoma. A number of later psychophysical investigations supported this theory. However, other histological studies and psychophysical investigations of glaucoma concluded that all nerve fiber populations, regardless of size, are damaged equally. This led to the redundancy theory (Figure 7.1 a and b) that states that all nerves are damaged equally in glaucoma.

Excess functional capacity or redundancy in some retinal systems means that the functional properties of these systems are not affected until the disease process is advanced. Additionally, those functional systems with reduced redundancy will yield functional loss early in the disease process. Despite the

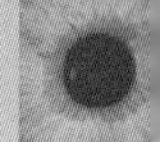

Cone population

Responses from B, G and R cones contribute to the normal achromatic response

B + G + R =

Threshold for normal achromatic pathway function

Damage to an area of retina leading to proportionately the same loss of B, G and R cones

Cone population

B + G + R =

Damage to the retina does not impair the function of the R and G pathways due to their redundancy. Less redundancy of the blue cones leads to functional impairment of the B pathway when the retina is damaged, but the normal function of the G and R pathways masks this impairment in the achromatic response, which remains normal

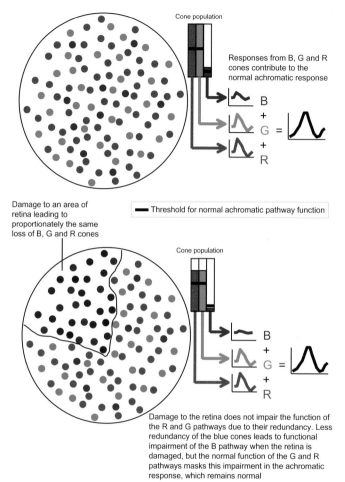

Figure 7.1 The redundancy theory

equivocal nature of the mechanism of glaucomatous damage, if a novel visual field test could be developed which is a selective measure of specific nerve fiber populations and retinal functional systems, damage to the visual pathway could be detected at an earlier stage than with conventional perimetry.

Short-wavelength automated perimetry

A number of disease processes, such as glaucoma and diabetes, yield foveal blue-yellow color vision deficiencies (triton) which occur in the early stages of the diseases. This observation led to the development of short-wavelength automated perimetry (SWAP) in the mid 1980s. In this method of visual field examination, the standard white background of the perimeter is replaced with a higher luminance yellow background. The spectral properties of the background saturate neural responses from the retinal processing pathways governing long-wavelength (red), medium-wavelength (green) and rod responses. The short-wavelength pathway can then be investigated using a blue stimulus. The wavelength of the stimulus (440 to 460 nm) corresponds to the maximum spectral sensitivity of the short-wavelength (blue) sensitive visual pathway and has a narrow bandwidth, so that the medium-wavelength system is not stimulated. Because the normal human visual system is relatively insensitive to the detection of blue light, and the narrow bandwidth of the stimulus reduces its transmission, the measurement or dynamic range of the perimeter is grossly reduced when compared to that for white light stimuli. Consequently, the visual field is investigated using a Goldmann Size V stimulus, in order to increase dynamic range and enhance spatial summation for detection of the stimulus. The Octopus and Humphrey perimeters are able to perform visual field examination using SWAP.

In the early 1990s a number of clinical investigations showed that glaucomatous visual field loss is evident in SWAP up to five years before it becomes manifest with conventional (achromatic) perimetry. Further studies showed that visual field progression is also in advance of standard perimetry. The ability of SWAP to detect visual field loss before it becomes apparent with achromatic perimetry can be explained by the selective damage or the redundancy theories. The nerve fibers of the parvocellular visual pathway possess a smaller diameter than those of the magnocellular pathway. But those nerves conveying short-

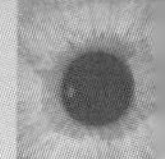

wavelength information possess a greater diameter than the medium- and long-wavelength fibers. It is therefore possible that short-wavelength fibers are damaged earlier in the glaucomatous disease process, yielding visual field defects before those detectable with achromatic perimetry, which stimulates all visual pathways equally. Alternatively, damage to the short-wavelength pathway can be explained by the redundancy theory. Blue cones, and therefore the retinal nerve fibers conveying short-wavelength spectral information, are fewer in number than green and red cones, accounting for approximately 15% of the total number of cones. The relative paucity of blue cones means that there is less redundancy in the short-wavelength sensitive pathway and, thus, if damage from glaucoma occurs equally to all visual pathways, the functional properties of the short-wavelength sensitive pathway will be impaired before those of the other spectral pathways (Figure 7.1).

The promise of these early research investigations prompted perimeter manufacturers to gather normative data for the development of statistical analysis packages for SWAP. However, SWAP has failed to gain widespread clinical usage. The primary reason for this is that the blue stimulus is absorbed by the ocular media (mostly the crystalline lens), which is a presents particular difficulties for evaluating the elderly population which is most at risk of developing glaucoma. The absorption of the stimulus by the ocular media results in gross variations in the normal height of the hill of vision. This, combined with the greater between-subject variability in normal subjects in SWAP, has confounded the statistical separation of focal from diffuse visual field loss, reducing the clinical viability of the test. Until the statistical evaluation of SWAP can be improved, it is unlikely to be adopted as a routine clinical investigation and so it is still largely confined to research investigations.

Flicker perimetry

At the same time SWAP was being developed, a number of other investigators developed a visual field investigation which was tuned to the functional properties visual pathway governed by cells of large diameter, namely the magnocellular pathway. A number of research investigations have shown that sensitivity to flicker is affected in a variety of eye diseases, including glaucoma, optic neuritis, retinitis pigmentosa and age-related macular degeneration. Flicker perimetry can be accomplished in two ways, critical fusion frequency (CFF) and temporal modulation perimetry (TMP). In CFF testing, the flicker contrast remains constant (usually close to 100% contrast) and the frequency of the flicker is varied. The threshold is estimated as the highest frequency at which the flicker can be detected. In TMP, the temporal frequency of flicker is fixed and the threshold is estimated as the minimum contrast necessary to detect the flicker. A number of clinical investigations have illustrated the clinical utility of flicker perimetry for the early detection of glaucoma.

Flicker perimetry in the form of CFF is commercially available with the Octopus series of perimeters. During the examination, Goldmann size III stimuli, flickering with a frequency between 1 and 50 Hz, are presented in a staircase strategy for a stimulus duration of one second. The patient has to decide if the stimulus is a constant light or a flickering one and press the response button if flicker is perceived. The advantage of flicker perimetry is that the stimulus is not particularly degraded by media opacity and refractive defocus, but making the decision whether the stimulus is constant or flickering is a difficult one, making the test prone to false positive errors.

Frequency doubling technology

Frequency doubling technology (FDT) is based on the rationale that a technique which measures a specific subset of ganglion cells might detect damage earlier than one which measures the entire retinal population. A sinusoidal grating of low spatial frequency (0.25 cycles per degree) which undergoes rapid counterphase flicker of 25 Hz appears to the viewer to have twice the spatial frequency (Fig 7.2).

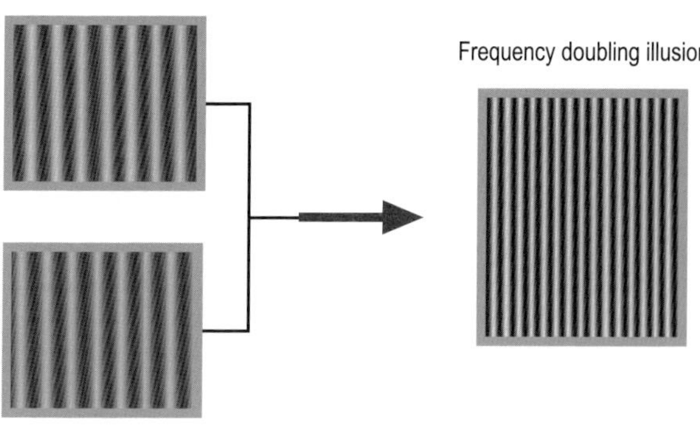

Figure 7.2 Frequency doubling illusion

This frequency doubling illusion is mediated by the magnocellular pathway and, more specifically, by a subset of cells called M_y cells. M_y cells possess a larger cell diameter than other magnocellular nerve fibers. In addition, they account for between 15 and 25% of the total number of magnocellular pathway fibers. Frequency doubling visual field loss associated with glaucoma can therefore be explained by both the selective damage and redundancy theories, in a similar manner to the explanation for the efficacy of SWAP.

The FDT instrument operates in a similar way to a perimeter. The patient views the instrument monocularly through an objective lens (Figure 7.3). Ametropia correction is thought to be less critical than for conventional visual field examination, as the FDT stimulus is less degraded by optical defocus. The manufacturers recommend that only magnitudes of ametropia over 7 D need to be corrected. At the standard testing distance, each square stimulus measures approximately 10-degrees and the central circle measures approximately 5-degrees. The frequency-doubling stimulus randomly presents itself at predetermined locations, for a maximum duration of 720 ms. FDT can be used in a suprathreshold screening or full threshold mode. Stimuli are presented in a modified binary search staircase procedure and the stimulus contrast is increased and decreased to estimate the threshold. Patient reliability is assessed using the same criteria as

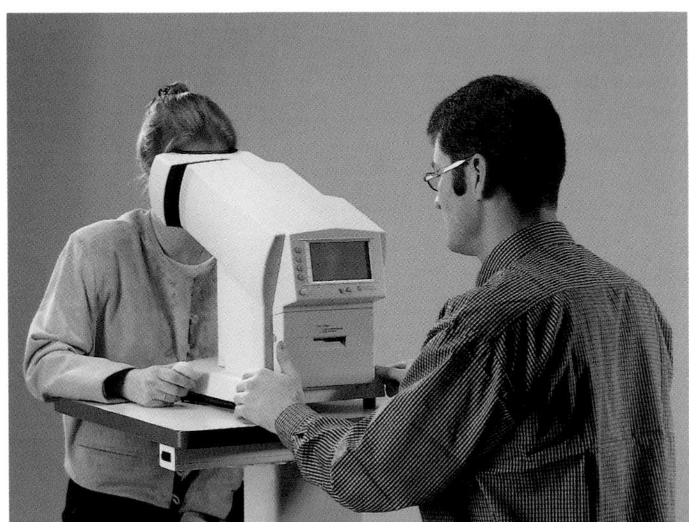

Figure 7.3 The Zeiss Humphrey FDT visual field instrument. Reproduced from Doshi and Harvey, *Investigative Techniques and Ocular Examination* (2003, Butterworth-Heinemann) with permission

in conventional perimetry (fixation losses, false positive and negative responses), although no camera is present to precisely align and monitor the patient's eye position. The statistical printout is similar to that of full threshold perimetry, with global indices sensitive for diffuse and focal visual field loss and total and pattern deviation probability plots.

A large number of comparative investigations of FDT and conventional perimetry have shown that FDT compares favorably in the separation of patients with early and severe glaucomatous visual field loss found with conventional perimetry. Some recent investigations have shown that FDT is a good predictor of glaucomatous damage occurring in ocular hypertensive patients. It would therefore appear that FDT is better than conventional perimetry for the detection of glaucomatous visual field loss, although further wide scale studies are still required. Investigations of test-retest variability, i.e. reproducibility in

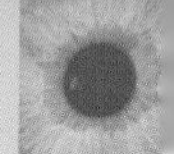

glaucoma, have shown that FDT does not increase as much with defect severity as it does with standard achromatic perimetry. This is advantageous for the assessment of visual field progression. In cataract, the mean deviation of FDT is affected in a similar way to achromatic perimetry. There is a significant correlation between the mean deviation of FDT and visual acuity. FDT is a sensitive tool for the rapid detection of neuro-ophthalmic visual field defects, although it does not appear to be able to accurately categorize hemianopic and quadrantanopic defects. FDT should not be considered, therefore, as a substitute for conventional perimetry, although it is a valuable adjunct to full threshold visual field examination. FDT has also been identified as being of potential use when evaluating patients with specific reading difficulties (dyslexia). Abnormalities in the magnocellular pathway have been implicated in this condition and appear to be detected using the frequency doubling illusion.

A recent development in FDT is the introduction of the Humphrey Matrix, which evaluates the visual field over 69 stimulus locations using 5 degree stimuli, which has a similar resolution to conventional achromatic visual field examination. Although initial research investigations suggest that the Humphrey Matrix correlates well with achromatic visual field examination, the nature of stimulus detection has not been investigated. The magnocellular pathway has very large receptive fields and it is questionable whether the stimulus size used is sufficient for M_y cell detection, or whether other detection mechanisms are involved.

Microperimetry

The Nidek MP-1 microperimeter is an innovative development in visual field measurement. The instrument is a hybrid between a fundus camera and a perimeter, capable of imaging the fundus whilst simultaneously measuring the visual field using either static or kinetic stimulus presentation. Stimuli are generated by means of an LCD display which is incorporated into the imaging system of the fundus camera. Landmark features on the fundus, such as blood

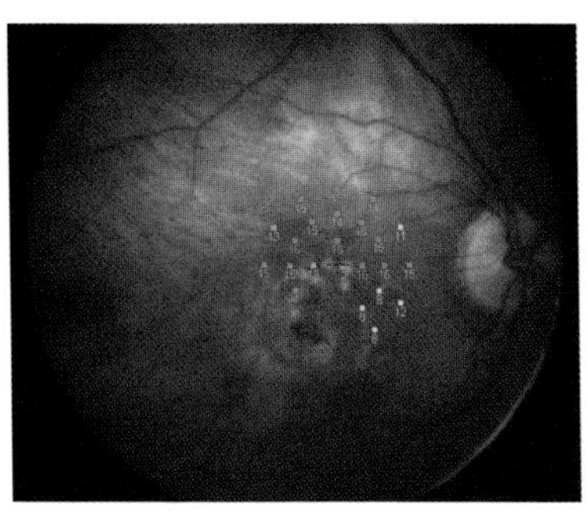

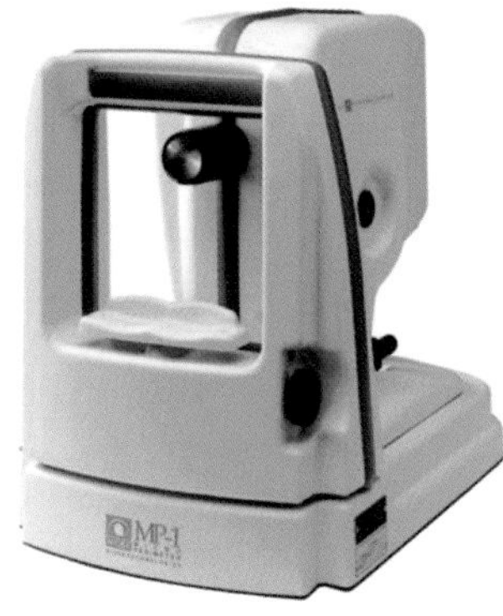

Figure 7.4 The Nidek MP1

vessels, are used to accurately track eye movements and precisely position light stimuli. The visual field results are superimposed over the fundus image, thus allowing for accurate mapping and monitoring of eye diseases ranging from optic nerve head disorders to maculopathy and more general diseases of the retina. The spatial resolution of visual field stimuli is much higher than can be obtained using conventional perimeters, making the instrument particularly useful for the investigation of maculopathy. The accurate and constant mapping of fixation enables the instrument to be used to train fixation for eccentric viewing in maculopathies which have damaged the foveal region (Figure 7.4)

Multifocal electroretinography

Clinical electrophysiology encompasses a variety of tests which measure the electrical responses of the brain and retina to visual and auditory stimuli. A recent advance in this field has been the development of multifocal electroretinography (mERG), commercially available as the VERIS (visual evoked response imaging system). This technique simultaneously records the electrical activity from 100 areas of the retina over an examination time of approximately seven minutes per eye. Thus, it is now possible to conduct a visual field examination whereby the results are determined objectively, rather than from the subjective responses of the patient.

The technique measures the potential difference between an active and a reference electrode. The active electrode is placed close to the cornea and the reference electrode near the outer canthus of the eye. Pupils are dilated prior to examination, which occurs with an appropriate near vision correction for the viewing distance of 30 cm. The mERG stimulus consists of a cathode ray tube monitor on which a series of hexagons are displayed. The hexagon size increases towards the visual field periphery, in accordance with the normal gradient of cone photoreceptors, in order that the electrical responses obtained are of approximately the same amplitude across the visual field. The patient views the screen and the hexagon pattern is rapidly flashed from black to white, according to a pseudo-random sequence, yielding on-off responses from the area of retina under examination. A large number of on-off responses are required in order to average the retinal responses. During the acquisition process the patient is not allowed to blink, as this generates large electrical signals which mask the retinal response. Consequently, data is gathered over equally spaced time segments, such that the total acquisition time is of the order of four minutes. The average signal for each segment is then amplified and band-passed filtered, in order to remove any extraneous electrical noise. The waveforms resulting from each hexagon can be analyzed in isolation or summed as rings and quadrants. The waveform of the first-order response has a biphasic nature. There is an initial negative deflection (N1) followed by a positive peak (P1). These deflections are thought to be comprised of similar components to a conventional full field ERG. Complex analysis of the waveform yields information about the signal generation properties of the inner and outer layers of the retina (Figure 7.5).

Although research investigations have identified changes in the mERG in glaucoma which may further our understanding of the disease process, its utility as a clinical test for early detection is currently unknown. The mERG procedure is the first time visual field investigation is able to be carried out objectively. But the examination procedures do not lend themselves to optometric practice, as they are complex to set up and, in some cases,

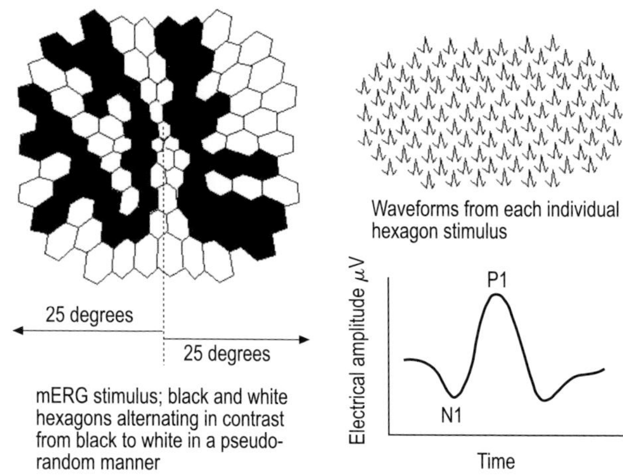

Figure 7.5 Multifocal ERG stimulus and response

difficult to complete as a high level of patient compliance is required. As a result, mERG investigations are likely to be confined to hospital practice.

Further Reading

Anderson, R.S. and O'Brien, C. (1997). Psychophysical evidence for a selective loss of M ganglion cells in glaucoma. *Vision Res.* **37**: 1079–1083.

Hood, D.C. (2000). Assessing Retinal Function with the Multifocal Technique. *Prog Ret Eye Res.* **19**: 607–646.

Johnson, C.A., Adams, A.J., Casson, E.J. and Brandt, J.D. (1993a). Blue-on-yellow perimetry can predict the development of glaucomatous visual field loss. *Arch. Ophthalmol.* **111**: 645–650.

Johnson, C.A., Adams, A.J., Casson, E.J. and Brandt, J.D. (1993b). Progression of early glaucomatous visual field loss as detected by blue-on-yellow and standard white-on-white automated perimetry. *Arch. Ophthalmol.* **111**: 651–565.

Landers, J.A., Goldberg, I. and Graham, S.L. (2003). Detection of early visual field loss in glaucoma using frequency-doubling perimetry and short-wavelength automated perimetry. *Arch Ophthalmol.* **121**: 1705–1710.

Morgan, J.E. (1994). Selective cell death in glaucoma: does it really occur? *Br. J. Ophthalmol.* **78**: 875–880.

Quigley, H.A., Addicks, E.M. and Green, W.R. (1982). Optic nerve damage in human glaucoma. Quantitative correlation of nerve fiber loss and visual field defect in glaucoma, ischemic neuropathy, papilledema, and toxic neuropathy. *Arch. Ophthalmol.* **100**: 135–146.

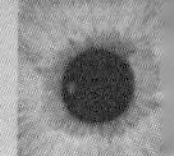

Quigley, H.A., Sanchez, R.M., Dunkelberger, G.R., L'Hernault, N.L. and Baginski, T.A. (1987). Chronic glaucoma selectively damages large optic nerve fibers. *Invest. Ophthalmol. Vis. Sci.* **28**: 913–920.

Quigley, H.A., Dunkelberger, G.R. and Green, W.R. (1989). Retinal ganglion cell atrophy correlated with automated perimetry in human eyes with glaucoma. *Am. J. Ophthalmol.* **107**: 453–464.

Spry, P.G.D. and Johnson, C.A. (2003). Within-test variability of frequency-doubling perimetry using a 24-2 test pattern. *J Glaucoma.* **11**: 315–320.

Wild, J.M., Cubbidge, R.P., Pacey, I.E. and Robinson, R. (1998). Statistical Aspects of the Normal Visual Field in Short-Wavelength Automated Perimetry. *Invest Ophthalmol Vis Sci.* **39**: 54–63.

Yoshiyama, K.K. and Johnson, C.A. (1997). Which method of flicker perimetry is most effective for detection of glaucomatous visual field loss? *Invest Ophthalmol Vis Sci.* **38**: 2270–2277.

8
Gross assessment of the visual field

Confrontation

Though the terms confrontation and gross perimetry are often used as synonyms, strictly speaking confrontation describes one of several "comparison" tests, whereas gross perimetry is the use of a target to measure the extent of the visual field and to map any large scotomas within the field. One form of confrontation involves the use of a target moved along an imaginary flat plane between, and perpendicular to, the gaze of the patient and the practitioner. This obviously will not allow the temporal extent of field to be measured, but will allow the practitioner to confirm that any areas they see can also be seen by the patient. One could also describe other tests as confrontation tests; for example, the presentation of two red targets to the hemifields of the patient to find out whether one of the targets is desaturated, or the use of a shiny coin in four quadrant of the field of one eye. Many confrontation tests are used by neurologists in investigating possible neurological lesions.

Gross perimetry

Gross perimetry describes the use of a handheld target held at a constant distance from the patient's eye (Figure 8.1) which, when brought in an arc from beyond their visual field boundary, allows them to announce when the target is first seen (the extent of field or boundary for that particular target size and color). When the target is moved further within their field to the central point of fixation it allows any large defect to be detected.

The choice of target dictates the extent of the isopter, just as with any kinetic assessment. A larger target will be seen at a greater eccentricity, while the isopter for a small target will be contracted. Similarly, a white target brought from beyond the field will be seen before a red target, which will itself be seen before a green target. In practice, though a small white target might be justifiable in terms of sensitivity, a red target is generally chosen as it will contrast better with typical wall coverings within the

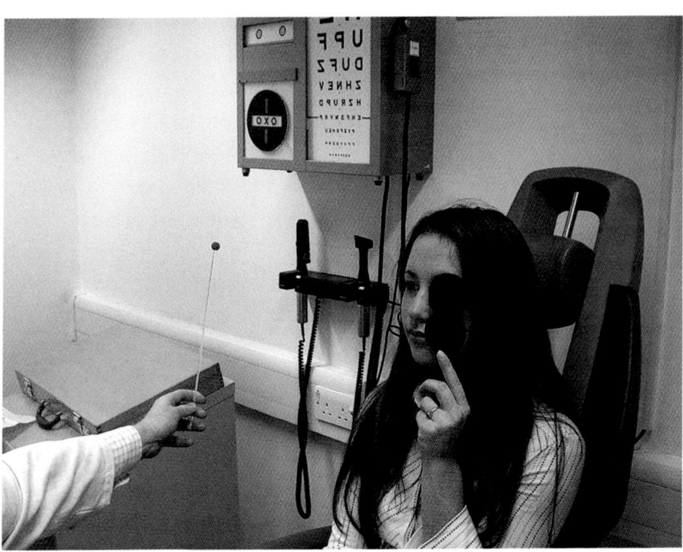

Figure 8.1 Gross perimetry

consulting room. To maintain some degree of correlation with a 5mm white target (typical for gross perimetry), a 15mm diameter red target may be used instead, its extra size counteracting the reduced sensitivity to red compared to white.

The extent of the absolute visual field is dependent upon the shape of the head of the patient, but it is important to remember that the extent of the temporal field is almost always greater than 90 degrees. Typical values are 100 degrees temporally, 75 degrees inferiorly, and 60 degrees nasally and superiorly. The last two are most patient dependent because of variable nose and brow size. To ensure a starting point beyond the visual field of the patient, therefore, the target should be held somewhat behind them for the temporal measurement.

Method

- As far as is possible in a cluttered consulting room, the surroundings should be as uniform and regular in color and contrast as is practicable. The patient should face the practitioner and occlude one eye. No correction should be worn by the patient. Though their hand may be used, this is not fully reliable, as many people cannot resist the urge to peak through small gaps between the fingers. An alternative would be for them to be given an occluder and helped to maintain this in front of one eye, such that the field of that eye is effectively excluded.

- Fixation shifts are one of the main causes of error in any field assessment technique and gross perimetry is no exception. The patient should be directed to stare with their uncovered eye, either at the bridge of the nose or into one of the practitioner's eyes and the practitioner should monitor a steady fixation throughout the test.
- The target should be held at about 35cm from the patient's eye and initially outside the field of view of the patient. The patient should then be told to say when they are first aware of the target as it is slowly but steadily moved around the imaginary arc (always at a constant distance from the eye). Once this position is reached (and a mental note made of it) the target should continue its passage to the center of the patient's view and the patient asked to report any point at which it disappears. If such is reported, the target may be moved about in this blind spot to find a rough outline of the area.
- This should be repeated in eight directions (superior, superior temporal, temporal, inferior temporal and so on). The same should then be carried out for the other eye. Though many practitioners speed up the technique and use only the four main meridians, this may result in a large quadrantanopia being missed.
- The most common error introduced in this method is the failure to maintain a constant distance from the patient's eye. The closer the target is to the eye, the less sensitive the test, as a small target movement will subtend a larger area of retina. Only very gross defects will be detected (so the assessment will have a high specificity). The further from the eye the target is, the more sensitive the test, but the more difficult the target

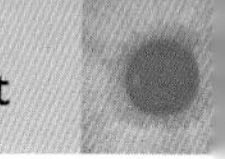

will be to spot for those without any defect (so specificity will reduce). 35cm is useful as it is usually comfortable for the practitioner, roughly equates to a bowl perimeter such as the Goldmann or the Humphrey Field Analyzer, and offers a reasonable balance of specificity and sensitivity (though both are not particularly high values due to the very gross nature of the test).

- Assuming the isopters equate roughly to typical values for the absolute visual field and there are no major defects within the field, the result should be noted as full on the record card. There are many perfectly innocuous situations where the field may be contracted; for example, the restricted superior field of an elderly patient due to ptosis. This should be noted on the record as such and not ignored.

As an examination technique, however, the above technique is insensitive, unless there is a gross constriction of the visual field, or a dense, widespread scotoma is present. The test has a low overall sensitivity of 63% for the detection of arcuate scotomas, altitudinal defects, visual field constriction, hemianopias and quadrantanopias. As a result, the test is a poor screening procedure and should only be used where there is no other means of visual field examination available.

The Amsler chart

The Amsler chart represents a simple method of assessing the quality of the central field of vision. The test includes several charts, the basic and most commonly used being a square white grid printed on a dull black background, comprising twenty rows and twenty columns of smaller squares (Figure 8.2).

When viewed at 28 cm, each square subtends one degree at the retina. The grid, therefore, is used to assess the field ten degrees either side of the fixation point when viewed monocularly (as should always be the case). It is, therefore, only possible to map out the physiological blind spot by directing the patient to view the nasal edge of the grid such that the blind spot

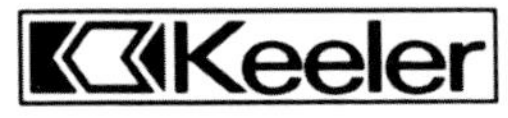

AMSLER RECORDING CHART

A replica of Chart No. 1, printed black on white for convenience of recording

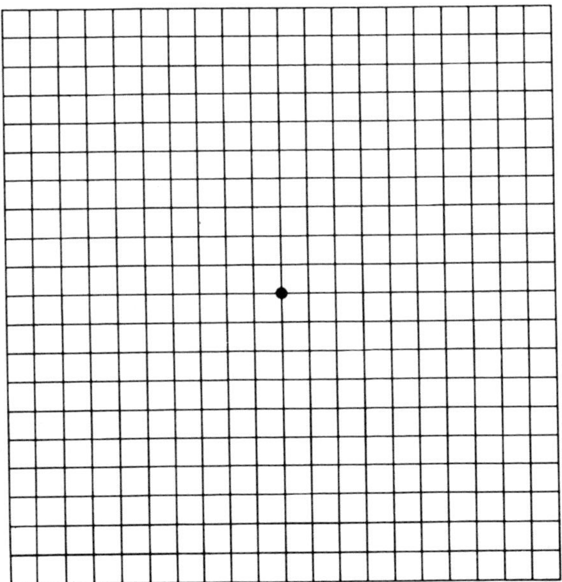

KEELER LIMITED
Clewer Hill Road, Windsor Berkshire SL4 4AA
Tel: (01753) 857177 Telex: 847565 Fax: (01753) 857817

CE

Ref. 2215-P-7057

Figure 8.2 Amsler grid

15 degrees temporal to this point falls onto the grid. Though rarely done, it is in theory possible to detect blind spot extension in, for example, myelinated nerve fibers around the disk or in early papilloedema. Typically, however, the grid is used to assess macular function.

Indications for its use include the following;

- Evidence of macular disturbance seen on ophthalmoscopy in either eye (if seen in just one eye, both eyes require investigation because of the bilateral nature of most macular diseases)
- Unexplainable loss of central visual acuity
- Reduction of acuity through a pinhole
- Symptoms of central visual disturbance, such as distortion
- History of systemic disease or, more commonly, drugs which may predispose to a maculopathy (such as tamoxifen or chloroquine). For the assessment of possible early toxic maculopathy, the red Amsler grid may be slightly more sensitive
- For the mapping of a central scotoma already detected. This is useful for monitoring any progression of a scotoma. For this assessment, the grid with diagonal cross lines is useful to encourage stable fixation. The patient should be asked to fixate upon the point where they imagine the center of the cross to be. In cases of poor performance with magnification, noting the position of the scotoma relative to the center is useful. A scotoma shifted towards the right of the field will have a greater impact upon the ability to scan from left to right when reading.
- History of poor photo stress recovery. Reports of persistent after-images after exposure to, for example, a flashlight or a difficulty in adapting to changes in ambient light levels may indicate early macular disease.

A simple procedure might be as follows:

- Correct the patient to adequately see the target at 28cm. Illumination should be good without constituting a glare source, and one eye should be occluded

- The patient should be directed to fixate upon the dot in the center of the grid. As poor fixation is perhaps the main source of error in any field assessment, this instruction cannot be repeated enough throughout the test
- While looking at the central target, the patient should report if any of the four corners of the grid are missing and, if so, the missing area should be shaded on the record sheet (a replica grid only in black on a white background)
- The patient should then report if any of the grid is missing and, if so, the position and size of the blind spot noted
- The patient should then report if any of the lines are wavy or distorted and again this recorded if found. If distorted, it is useful to note if the distortion is static (as might be the case with an old atrophic scar or a heavy concentration of drusen around the fovea) or moving or shimmering. The latter, described as metamorphopsia, might be indicative of an active exudative process (such as prior to choroidal neovascularisation) and might warrant an urgent referral

In cases where one eye has already suffered macular disease, or where there is evidence of macular disturbance yet to affect vision, many practitioners give a copy of the grid to the patient, who may then self-monitor their central field on a regular basis at home and in the knowledge that they must report any new disturbance they might detect.

Further Reading

Marmor, M.F. (2000). A brief history of macular grids: From Thomas Reid to Edvard Munch and Marc Amsler. *Surv Ophthalmol.* **44**: 343–353.

Shahinfar, S., Johnson, L.N., Madsen, R.W. (1995). Confrontation visual-field loss as a function of decibel sensitivity loss on automated static perimetry – implications on the accuracy of confrontation visual-field testing. *Ophthalmology.* **102**: 872–877.

9 Characteristics of glaucomatous field loss

Automated perimetry is one of the most useful clinical tools for diagnosing and monitoring glaucoma in clinical practice. Although glaucomatous defects can occur anywhere in the visual field, clinical testing regimes concentrate on visual field changes in the central thirty degrees eccentricity from fixation. The arrangement of the retinal nerve fibers causes characteristic visual field defects as nerve fiber bundles become affected by the disease process.

Diffuse visual field loss

A number of research reports have suggested that one of the earliest changes in the visual field in glaucoma is a mild, generalized reduction in sensitivity across the visual field, which is thought to derive from diffuse loss of retinal nerve fibers throughout the optic nerve. Such loss is only clinically detectable using automated full threshold static perimetry, but is often difficult to define conclusively, especially as other factors, such as media opacity and pupil miosis can also give rise to a generalized reduction in sensitivity. Consequently, a generalized reduction in visual field sensitivity should be considered with other clinical risk factors when arriving at a diagnosis of glaucoma.

Focal visual field loss

Typically, the earliest change in the visual field resulting from glaucoma manifests as small areas of focal loss in the paracentral visual field (Figure 9.1). Most commonly, these defects appear in the superior nasal aspect of the visual field. Since these from defects arise damage of nerve fiber bundles in the retina, their shape reflects their anatomical configuration and therefore respect the horizontal raphé. One or more areas of paracentral focal visual field loss may be present and can often be detected ophthalmoscopically as nerve fiber bundle defects. As glaucoma progresses, enlargement of paracentral scotomas leads to the formation of continuous areas of focal loss. These defects mimic

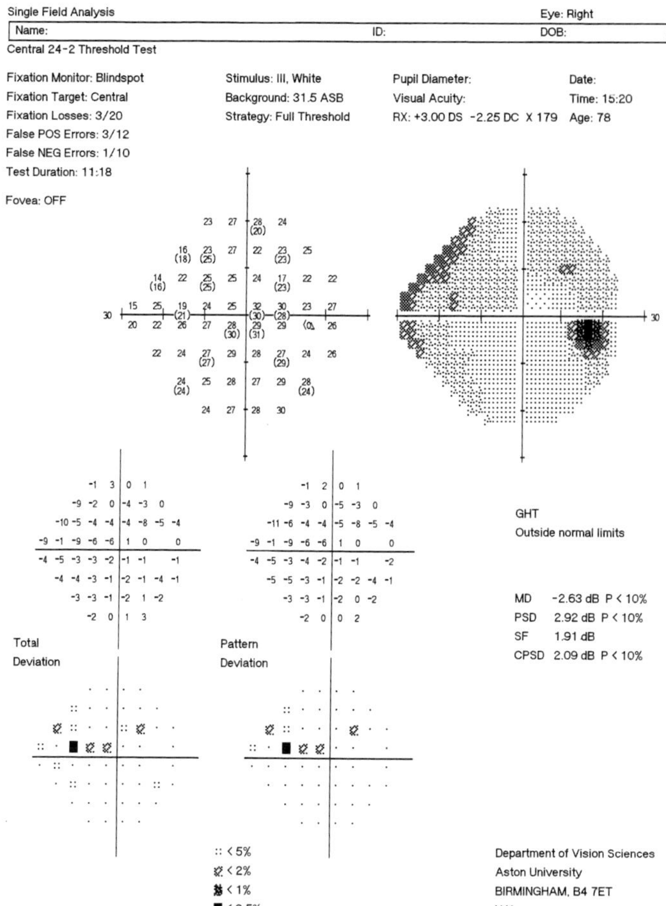

Figure 9.1 Nasal step

the course of the retinal nerve fibers and are termed arcuate scotomas. They may take many years to develop. Because arcuate scotomas are most commonly found in the superior hemifield, their termination at the horizontal midline leads to an area in the nasal visual field which has normal sensitivity on one side of the horizontal midline and reduced sensitivity on the other. When this occurs, there is said to be a nasal step (Figure 9.2). Nasal steps may also arise due to the formation of paracentral scotomas along the horizontal midline. They can occasionally be seen in a normal visual field, but if the step extends horizontally more than approximately five degrees, it should be considered as

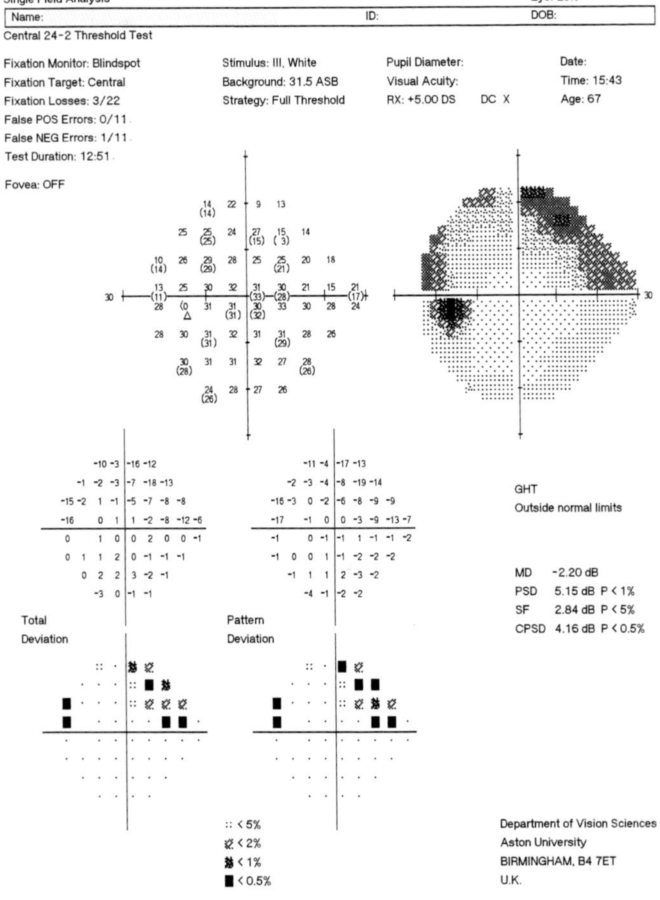

Figure 9.2 Superior arcuate defect

a pathological visual field. As glaucoma becomes more advanced, large arcuate scotomas may form in the superior and inferior visual fields (Figure 9.3). If these scotomas are symmetrical, they ultimately may lead to the formation of a ring scotoma. In the end stages of glaucoma only a small circular area of normal visual field sensitivity remains around fixation.

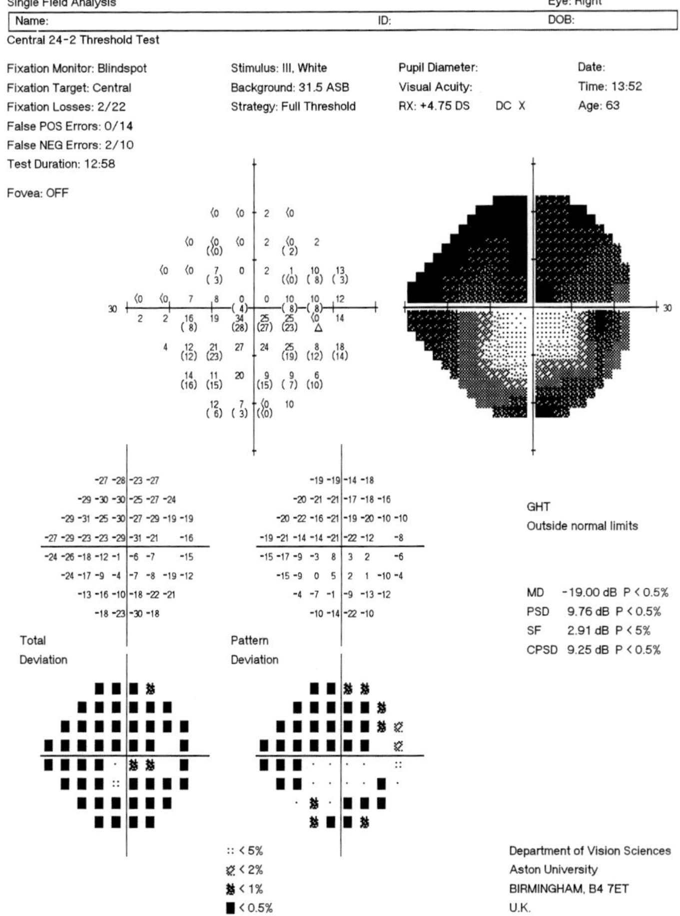

Figure 9.3 Advanced glaucoma loss

Visual field differences between high-tension and normal-tension glaucoma

Glaucoma is considered as an umbrella of disease states which produce characteristic visual field defects. In glaucoma where the intra-ocular pressure is high (HTG) and glaucoma where the intra-ocular pressure is normal (NTG) there are often perceived differences in the development of visual field defects. The superior visual field is preferentially affected in NTG, with defects appearing closer to fixation than in patients with HTG.

Classification of glaucomatous visual field loss

In quantitative suprathreshold visual field testing, the examiner should consider visual field defects in the paracentral region and in the peripheral nasal field along the horizontal midline as clinically significant, particularly if they occur in clusters of three or more adjacent stimulus locations. As with all types of perimetry, such defects should be repeatable on at least two consecutive occasions. In full threshold perimetry, statistical analysis algorithms aid the practitioner in diagnosis. The Glaucoma Hemifield Test (see Chapter 6) is optimized for the detection of glaucomatous visual field loss. The pattern deviation probability plot may be used to identify repeatable clusters probability in locations consistent with glaucoma (either three locations depressed at a level of statistical significance of $P < 5\%$ or one location depressed at $P < 1\%$). The focal loss global indices may also aid diagnosis; a PSD or CPSD at a $P < 5\%$ should be considered as clinically significant.

Large scale epidemiology studies of glaucoma and its treatment have been underway at various locations around the world for a number of years. Such studies need to be able to quantify glaucomatous visual field loss precisely and have developed scoring systems in order to facilitate the analysis of glaucomatous visual field progression. Of particular note is the Advanced

Glaucoma Intervention Study (AGIS) in the USA. A classification method for grading the status of glaucomatous visual fields derived using the Humphrey Field Analyzer 24-2 program has been developed and is particularly useful for making clinical judgements in practice. A scoring system ranging from 0 to 20 classifies visual fields from normal to end-stage glaucoma.

Further reading

Henson, D.B., Artes, P.H. and Chauhan, B.C. (1999). Diffuse loss of sensitivity in early glaucoma. *Invest Ophthalmol Vis Sci.* **40**: 3147–3151.

Samuelson, T.W. and Spaeth, G.L. (1993). Focal and diffuse visual field defects: their relationship with intra-ocular pressure. *Ophthalmic Surg.* **24**: 519–525.

Åsman, P. and Heijl, A. (1992). The Glaucoma hemifield test. Automated visual field evaluation. *Arch Ophthalmol.* **110**: 812–819.

AGIS Investigators (1994). The Advanced Glaucoma Intervention Study. 2. Visual field test scoring and reliability. *Ophthalmology.* **101**: 1445–1455.

10 Glossary of terminology

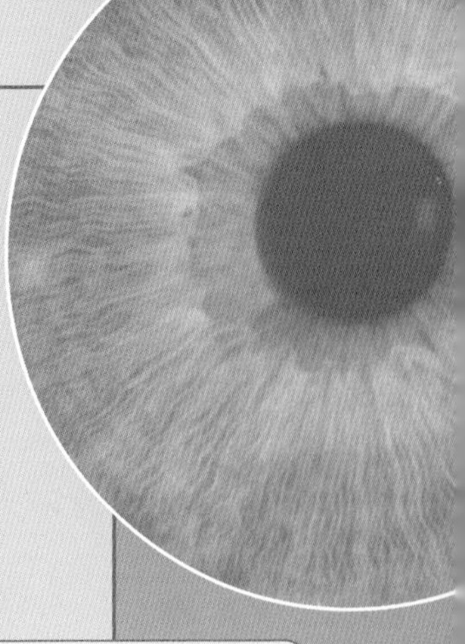

Depression

Overall reduction in retinal sensitivity to light stimuli, as might occur with cataract.

Contraction

Reduction in the extent of the field (and so distance of isopters from fixation), as might occur in retinitis pigmentosa or later stage glaucoma.

Focal loss

Reduction of the visual field at a specific area within the overall field.

Relative scotoma

A field defect representing a reduction in retinal sensitivity to light compared to the surrounding retina.

Absolute scotoma

An area of the field with no light perception, so representing a blind spot within the field.

Centrocaecal defect

A loss of the field extending nasally from the blind spot, resulting from selective damage to the papillomacular bundle. This may occur subsequent to, for example, toxic damage.

Nasal step

A difference in retinal sensitivity above and below the horizontal midline in the nasal field. This is a characteristic defect in early glaucoma.

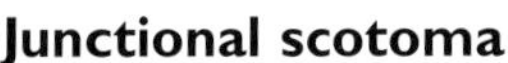

Junctional scotoma

A defect showing respect of the vertical midline as typical, due to damage to the visual pathway at the chiasma or post-chiasmal tissues. A lesion immediately anterior to the chiasma in the optic nerve by, for example, a meningioma, will affect inferior nasal fibers from the contralateral eye (anterior knee of Wilbrand) will also cause a junctional defect.

Congruence

This represents similarity in the shape of the field defect present in each eye; the more similar, the greater the congruence. Congruence increases after the reprocessing of fibers that takes place in the lateral geniculate nuclei.

Gradient adaptation

The incorporation into a field analyzer of a feature that accommodates for the decreasing sensitivity of the retina and enlargement of receptive field size towards the periphery of the cornea. This might be brighter or larger stimuli towards the peripheral field.

Full threshold

Stimuli are presented at a level at which the viewer is just able to perceive them. The stimulus brightness is usually specified in decibel units (dB) or as a log unit. The two are related by a factor of 10, 1 log unit equals 10dB.

Suprathreshold

Stimuli are presented at a brightness level above threshold by a specified amount.

Algorithm

In a generic sense, this term may be applied to any set of rules that outlines a sequence of actions undertaken to solve a problem. The rules are precise and so may be carried out automatically. In field screening, the algorithm normally describes the settings a machine will operate in terms of stimulus brightness and location to establish sensitivity data for specified locations in the visual field.

Up–down staircase thresholding

The method commonly used to establish threshold, whereby perceived stimuli are succeeded at the same location by fainter stimuli, and non-perceived stimuli followed by brighter ones.

Crossing or reversal of threshold

The situation in which a stimulus crosses from seen to unseen or vice versa. Typically, a double-crossing technique may be used whereby the stimulus brightness is reduced until no longer seen (first crossing or single reversal) and then increased until seen again (second crossing or double reversal).

A 4-2dB algorithm

A program in which there is a change in stimulus brightness in 4dB steps until the first reversal is achieved and then in 2dB steps until second reversal is reached.

SITA

This stands for the Swedish interactive thresholding algorithm, and is incorporated as an option in Humphrey Field Analysers, 700 series onwards. It was designed as an attempt to decrease the time taken for a traditional staircase method assessment (a 4-2dB algorithm typically takes 15 minutes) and yet maintain good sensitivity in glaucoma detection. Time is reduced in several ways as the algorithm specifies the appropriate stimulus

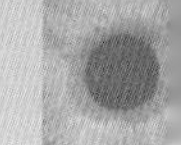

brightness to be presented at each point, may monitor the time of response to adopt appropriate subsequent presentations and is able to stop once sufficient information has been taken. The presentation of stimuli at levels around that at which 50 per cent are seen greatly reduces the speed of testing. So, by better pacing of the test, and the useful interpretation of false positives and false negatives, the SITA appears to correlate well with standard perimetric assessment, but in less time. The reduced timing is likely to help the accuracy of response.

Heijl–Krakau technique

A method of monitoring fixation throughout a field assessment by projecting a stimulus to an assumed location of the blind spot. If fixation is not present, the patient will respond to this stimulus and the machine will note the number of errors. The technique relies on an estimate of the exact location of the optic disk, and is thus open to error.

Gaze-tracking

As opposed to individual blind-spot assessment at specified times during assessment, often primarily at the beginning of the test, gaze tracking allows a continual assessment of fixation throughout by monitoring the relative positions of every stimulus presented.

False negative

Usually used to describe a stimulus presented at a specified increased brightness to a previously seen point that is now not seen. For example, in a FASTPAC screening, a false negative will be recorded when a seen point is then missed when presented at 9dB brighter.

False positive

Typically describes the point at which a patient responds to a stimulus that was not presented. This usually occurs during pauses incorporated into the program when no stimuli are presented, to allow for some assessment of accuracy of response.

Step-by-step fields interpretation

The following represents a noteform checklist that summarizes the clues that allow field interpretation to be localized to a specific lesion site.

- One eye only – most likely pre-chiasmal (except where affecting anterior knee of Wilbrand)
- Respects horizontal – retinal
- Respects vertical – chiasmal or post-chiasmal
- Heteronymous – chiasmal
- Homonymous – post-chiasmal
- Homonymous and congruent – post-lgn
- Homonymous and incongruent – likely tract
- Homonymous and superior quad – likely Meyer's loop (temporal lobe)
- Homonymous hemianopia – likely occipital (with macular sparing)
- Pre-LGN – pupil reflexes affected
- Tract/chiasmal – bilateral optic atrophy
- Pre-chiasmal – unilateral optic atrophy

Supportive assessment

- Ophthalmoscopy – reveals retinal abnormalities
- Pupils – reveals pre-LGN lesions
- Monocular color vision – reveals retinal abnormalities and acquired defects

Index

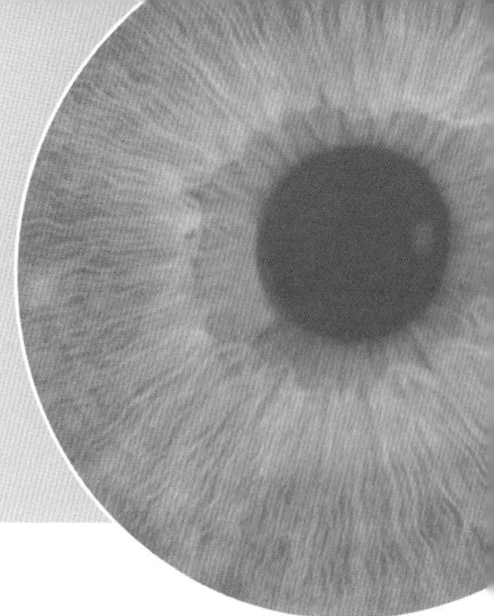

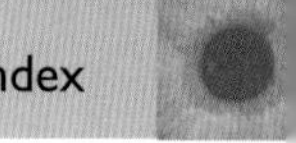

T

U

V

Z